T0261387

Handbook of Hypnotic Inductions

GEORGE GAFNER, CISW
SONJA BENSON, PH.D.

W.W. Norton & Company
New York • London

Composition by Ken Gross
Manufacturing by Haddon Craftsmen

Library of Congress Cataloging-in-Publication Data

Gafner, George, 1947–
   Handbook of hypnotic inductions / George Gafner, Sonja Benson.
      p.   cm.
   "A Norton professional book."
   Includes bibliographical references and index.
   ISBN 0-393-70324-X
   1. Hypnotism—Therapeutic use—Handbooks, manuals, etc.
I. Benson, Sonja, 1968–   II. Title.

RC495.G27   2000
615.8'512–dc21   99-053494

W. W. Norton & Company, Inc., 500 Fifth Avenue, New York, NY 10110
www.wwnorton.com

W.W. Norton & Company, Ltd., 10 Coptic Street, London WC1A 1PU

6 7 8 9 0

Contents

Introduction

The inductions in this book are intended to bolster the hypnotherapy repertoires of masters-level and above practitioners who treat anxiety disorders, mood disorders, chronic pain, and other health and mental health problems. This work had its genesis in the hypnotherapy training groups at the Tucson (Arizona) Veterans Affairs Medical Center. I (SB) was a psychology intern at the Tucson V.A. in the mid-1990s, and I now have my own clinical practice at the Phoenix V.A. Medical Center. In addition, I have a private clinical practice and teach a psychology course at a local college. I (GG) continue to conduct this training along with Bob Hall, Ph.D., who specializes in health psychology. In our training groups members begin immediately to learn about hypnotic phenomena and the principles of hypnotherapy by experiencing trance both as operators and subjects. Group members then gradually progress to various applications of hypnotherapy in their respective clinical rotations. As we began this training in the mid-1980s, we discovered a dearth of useful hypnotic

inductions and accordingly we began to add our own scripted hypnotic inductions to the ones culled from books and training manuals.

Hypnotherapists are first and foremost *therapists*, with requisite
education and training, initially in a specific discipline and in psychotherapy, and subsequently in hypnosis. As therapists, they employ hypnotherapy as one of several methods in treating clients. In
our own practices we use hypnotherapy to a large extent, but we also
rely on cognitive-behavioral, solution-focused, strategic, and other
approaches with individuals, couples, and families. In general, we
practice brief therapy, but we recognize that some people require
long-term support. We believe that the fundamental job of the therapist is to discover or stimulate resources already possessed by the
client. Such resources are sometimes unconscious and are often best
accessed through hypnosis, which has been defined in a host of
ways, including intensely focused attention, heightened state of
receptivity or responsiveness, influenced communication, or controlled dissociation. In addition to using those descriptions, we may
define it to clients as "controlled imagination," an ability possessed
by all people but to varying degrees. Zeig (1991) states that hypnosis
is an experience *elicited* from within, not induced from without. The
task of the therapist is to help people utilize this natural ability to
solve the problems they bring to therapy. In other words, the therapist establishes a climate for change, but the motive force comes
from the client (Zeig, 1991).

We are guided by the work of Milton H. Erickson and those who
have built upon his foundation for influencing behavior change—
Stephen Gilligan, Jay Haley, D. Corydon Hammond, Bill O'Hanlon,
Stephen and Carol Lankton, Ernest L. Rossi, Jeffrey K. Zeig, Brent
Geary, and so many others. Erickson, the consummate optimist, had
a future orientation and believed that, although the past cannot be
changed, one's views and interpretations of it can be (Beahrs, 1971).
We believe that many clients' resources are stimulated by a hypnotherapeutic approach that is permissive, indirect, metaphorical,
and nonauthoritarian. Clients experience this approach as respectful
and refreshing. They are able to recognize that the therapist is but a
guide whose job is to bring out the strengths they already own. Nevertheless, since some clients may expect a directive and authoritarian approach, we have included some inductions of that type.

Most practitioners consider a typical session of hypnotherapy to consist of three basic parts: the induction, deepening, and therapy. Enveloping this framework are a few minutes of talking at the beginning of the hour and a debriefing at the end. For example, after the client reports on current symptoms, the therapist and client together set an agenda that includes a review of overall goals as well as specific goals for the day. Following induction and deepening, they enter the therapeutic portion of the session. For example, for clients who want to learn pain management, the therapist may offer direct suggestions for decreasing pain, transfer pain to a more manageable location through a metaphor or story, or use a visualization technique to imagine the pain scale moving to a more comfortable level. For other clients, therapeutic components may include ego-strengthening, problem-solving, abreactive work, management of anxiety, or numerous other applications.

The foundation and most essential aspect of the trance process is the induction. The induction—along with deepening—produces relaxation, builds trust and rapport, and stimulates the client's imagination. The induction is both the vehicle and the route to the therapeutic end. We liken the induction to an ocean liner and the therapy component to an island. Without a good induction there is little chance of reaching the island. In other words, without a good induction there can be no good hypnotherapy.

In this book we offer a variety of inductions in five main categories: conversational, embedded-meaning, confusional, directive, and appropriate for children. We believe that teaching of the deepening portion of trancework in workshops and in training manuals has been woefully mundane, traditional, and lacking in imagination. As a bridge between induction and therapy, the deepening should both enhance the induction and *set up* the therapy component. With each induction we try to demonstrate the virtually limitless and highly purposeful possibilities that practitioners can explore to enhance the trancework process.

The examples selected for induction and deepening range from basic to complex. In addition to sharing these examples, we highlight key concepts and principles of hypnotherapy. Most of all, we wish to stimulate readers to develop their own inductions to meet the particular needs of their clients. The inductions in this book have been used hundreds if not thousands of times with clients who have a variety of clinical problems. Through practice we all develop facility and confidence, and our confidence in hypnotherapy is immediately conveyed to our clients.

We are members of the American Society of Clinical Hypnosis (ASCH) and have benefited immensely from training provided by the Milton H. Erickson Foundation in Phoenix, Arizona. We encourage you to explore training and membership opportunities in ASCH, a Milton H. Erickson society in your state or country, or a similar body. These are listed at the end of the book, along with references on which we have drawn—resources that we hope you, too, will read and enjoy.

ACKNOWLEDGMENTS

Our thanks to our families for their understanding and support, to Susan Munro at Norton for opening the door, to Monica Friedman for her superb editorial assistance, and to Dr. Bob Hall for his patience and wisdom. "Rocket Man," you've come a long way from Des Moines . . .

Handbook of Hypnotic Inductions

1

Essential Considerations
in Hypnotherapy

INTRODUCING THE CLIENT TO TRANCEWORK

Let us imagine meeting with a client, Guillermo, for the first time. He is a 33-year-old Hispanic male who is referred for anxiety. Guillermo, who is seen at a satellite clinic of the Phoenix Veterans Affairs Medical Center, served uneventfully in the Air Force ten years ago. He is curious about hypnosis but has some reservations about losing control, as he once witnessed stage hypnosis at a comedy club where people on stage "did a bunch of weird things." Nevertheless, Guillermo is eager to do something to manage his anxiety, and he has declined the offer of medications from his physician.

I (SB) tell Guillermo that usually no hypnosis is done during the first session because I first want to learn more about him so that I will be in a better position to help him. During the first appointment I try to accomplish these things: take a history that emphasizes the social context of the presenting problem, dispel negative notions about hypnosis, perhaps give the client information to read about hypnosis, answer any questions, elicit naturalistic trance experiences, educate the client about trancework, and overall, build expectancy. During the first session I will also do any other assessment that is indicated.

ADDRESSING ISSUES OF CONTROL

Clients new to psychotherapy are likely to be anxious, apprehensive, and understandably reluctant to reveal personal information to the therapist. We are always respectful of such hesitancy, which clients invariably signal nonverbally long before they express it in words. We often say something like, "Tell me only what is necessary to have me help you now." Such a statement communicates both restraint and permission, along with the implication that they will indeed open up more in the future.

In hypnotherapy, there are several things the therapist may do to enhance clients' feelings of control. We may make an attempt at humor, for example, "Guillermo, if you quack like a duck on command, you'll be the first client I've ever had who has done so." We might also reframe cautiousness as something protective and helpful: "It's okay to hold back, that's perfectly natural" or, "People in trance will reveal only what they want to." A very economical way to communicate all these things is by way of metaphor, for example, "Guillermo, in trance you will experience many interesting things, but *you are always in the driver's seat*." It is vital that the therapist thoroughly address issues of control; otherwise clients may not return for another session. Our general rule of thumb is: the more psychopathology there is, the slower we go.

During the first session of hypnotherapy, we usually lead clients into trance for a minute or two, bring them out of trance, and then resume hypnosis. We routinely bring very apprehensive clients in and out of trance several times. In addition to amplifying their self-control, this often causes them to go deeper into trance with each experience.

THE "HIDDEN OBSERVER"

Another way to enhance clients' feeling of control is to educate about what they may experience in trance. One common phenomenon is what Hilgard (1968) called the *hidden observer*. This may be experienced in various ways. Age-regressed clients may experience themselves simultaneously as a child and as an adult. Others may experience a part of themselves contemplating the therapist's words while another part notices internal phenomena such as a change in heart rate. Others may experience doubt or unwillingness to comply with a suggestion for hand levitation while watching their right hand slowly and involuntarily move upward. To Guillermo, I may say, "You will experience any number of things internally, privately, and a part of you may at the same time wonder 'How can this be happening?' One client, one time, described it as a little man sitting there on his shoulder. It's interesting how two or more things can go on at the same time, almost like driving a car, where your hands do one thing, your feet another, and you're paying attention to traffic and maybe listening to the radio—all at the same time."

Interns in our training groups encounter this phenomenon in yet a different way. As they are experiencing trance as a subject, a part of them—sometimes a large part—struggles to not let go, simply because they want to pay attention to technique and process. Videotaping the experience may help them enter the experience more fully. Also, clinicians occasionally report the presence of the hidden observer during their work with clients, as therapists cannot help but go into at least a mild depth of trance themselves.

ELICITING NATURALISTIC TRANCE EXPERIENCE

As part of the orientation, we elicit naturally occurring trance experiences, letting clients know that what they are about to experience is not much different from other times they have been in a "natural" trance. We offer examples like listening to music, reading a good book, or when "you become absorbed in something, perhaps a long and boring drive, and time seems to pass slowly, or quickly, a minute might seem like an hour, or an hour like a minute, and you simply lose track of time." In Guillermo's case, he was able to cite several naturally occurring trance experiences, including driving home from work, playing tennis on weekends, and lulling his young daughter to sleep with a bedtime story.

INTRODUCING UNCONSCIOUS PROCESS

When the word *unconscious* is mentioned, some clients equate the term with orthodox psychoanalysis and believe that we are talking about a cauldron of untamed aggressive impulses that should be suppressed. Many clients are relieved to learn that among Ericksonians the unconscious is seen as a potent constructive force for life and growth. We explain to clients that successful living requires a smooth coordination between the unconscious mind and conscious awareness (Beahrs, 1971). We educate clients about the unconscious mind, telling them that this part of their mind is like the big part of the iceberg underneath the water, watchful and waiting, a repository of resources that can be utilized "now when you need them the most." We tell them that the hypnotherapist is but a guide to help them access and make use of their natural talents and abilities.

We might mention dreaming as an example of unconscious functioning or say, "Certainly you've watched young children playing, how everything is *imagination . . . fascination . . .* they're not thinking about paying the bills or getting the muffler fixed." We also tell them how we will be using stories, metaphors, confusion, and similar devices "to get in underneath the radar," which they invariably understand and come to appreciate. We tell them, "You might wonder, 'Why is she saying *that*?' Then recall that everything I say is to help you with your problem." We might also tell clients that the unconscious mind is seen as protective in that it only embraces suggestions that are acceptable to it at any given time.

After asking if they are right-handed or left-handed, which is important to know for the arm catalepsy induction and for ideomotor signaling, we ask, "Okay, so you're right-handed, but are you right-thumbed or left-thumbed?" Usually they respond with, "What?" and we say, "Well, let's see which you are. Please do this," and they are asked to interclasp their fingers behind their head and then bring the hands forward to their lap. If the left thumb is on top, we say, "See—you're left-thumbed—I bet you didn't know that." This is explained as unconscious process, "where things just happen all by themselves, not much different from daydreaming, or driving a car, where your feet and hands work seemingly all by themselves."

PREVIOUS EXPERIENCE WITH TRANCEWORK THAT WAS POSITIVE

Some clients have had previous experience with trancework. They might call it meditation, guided imagery, stress management exercises, or any number of things that induced trance. If their experience was positive, it is important to find out what was useful, so we can build on that experience. For example, if Guillermo reveals, "The therapist just had me sit back and close my eyes and afterward my hands felt very numb and it was a pleasant experience," we note that information so that we can incorporate it into the induction. Similar useful information is contained in statements such as, "Years ago I tried Transcendental Meditation and my mind just drifted off," or "When I go to church I lose myself in a hymn," or "When I pray I lose track of time altogether."

Information such as this may be directly utilized in an induction, for example, "Guillermo, you know what it's like to let those eyes gently close, and once they close, you can imagine that numbness beginning to develop in your hands." Utilization can also be employed in a more general and indirect fashion: "Guillermo, like all people, you've had pleasant experiences in the past when your mind just drifted off . . . losing yourself in an enjoyable activity . . . when keeping track of time actually becomes rather difficult to do. . . . "

PREVIOUS EXPERIENCE WITH TRANCEWORK THAT WAS NEGATIVE

Many clients who have had a negative experience in the past will decline when hypnotherapy is first offered. Others may agree to participate but then later passively resist the process. If you spend some time discovering the basis of their beliefs, you might be able to successfully dispel these negative notions. Other clients, though, equate hypnosis and hypnotherapy with brainwashing or mind control or see it as contrary to their religious beliefs. With these clients we often do not pursue trancework.

Some people may have attended a show featuring stage hypnosis at a county fair or in a night club and witnessed people doing outlandish behavior on command. We usually tell clients who relate such experiences that what they saw was indeed hypnosis, but hypnosis done for entertainment. Clinical hypnosis, on the other hand, is serious and done to help people with their problems.

Cheek (1994) proposed that some clients' resistance to trancework has its roots in an early negative experience that can be accessed only on the unconscious level. To access this event the therapist asks questions of the unconscious mind, which responds through ideomotor movements such as finger signals.

SEEDING

Seeding involves mentioning something in different ways early on so that later, when it is mentioned again, the target is activated by the earlier "seed." This process may be viewed as "priming the pump." With anxious clients, for example, you may seed *slowing down* in several ways: by mentioning at the outset of the session that traffic was especially *slow* driving to work today; nonverbally by *slowly* getting up from your desk to retrieve your coffee cup; or by *slowing down* your speech or rate of breathing. Later on, during formal trancework, when you refer to *slowing down* in a story about driving down a road, the client is more likely to accept the suggestion (Zeig, 1990). Since this is a vital technique, we employ it liberally in this book. Geary (1994) makes an important distinction between seeding and suggestion, pointing out that with seeding there is always follow-up.

COMMUNICATING IN TRANCE: FACILITATING "THE DANCE"

Imagine that you are attending a social occasion at which people are dancing. You and your partner pay close attention to each other, each anticipating and responding to the other's movements. You understand each other and move in unison as you dance together.

Communication in hypnotherapy is much like a dance. While speaking to the client, the therapist simultaneously pays close attention to such things as a subtle postural shift, a brief eye flutter, a slight reddening in the cheeks, or the flaring of one nostril. The therapist then gives a suggestion. Perhaps he or she induces heaviness or some other feeling in the hands or asks the client to imagine something, such as walking down a staircase as part of deepening, or some time in the past when he or she experienced confidence. How does the therapist verify that the client has experienced these things? There are several ways, but they all involved asking.

"The dance" occurs when therapist and client can communicate back and forth. A good way to start is to ask for a head nod, e.g., "When you begin to detect a numbness or tingling, lightness or heaviness, or some other interesting sensation developing in one of those hands, let me know by nodding your head." You can also say, "Tell me with your words," although speaking has a tendency to lighten the client's trance.

With most clients we establish ideomotor finger signals early in therapy. Once in trance, we ask them to choose, on their dominant hand, a *yes* finger, a *no* finger, and an *I-don't know/not-ready-to-answer-yet* finger. As much of the trancework is on an unconscious level, we direct questions to the unconscious mind, e.g., "I want to ask a question of your unconscious mind. When you are ready to go deep into trance, you will know and I will know because one of your fingers will twitch and develop a lightness all its own and move up into the air." For the purposes of induction and deepening, the *yes* finger will be employed most in this book. For a detailed discussion of the application of finger signals, see Rossi and Cheek (1988).

UTILILIZATION

Also referred to as Ericksonian utilization, this is both a principle and a concept. It is also a standard approach for practitioners of the "new hypnosis," whose application requires specific techniques. At first blush, utilization appears simple, but many therapists become confused when they are unable to decide what behavior, if any, should be utilized.

A woman named Deb told me she hired a landscaper to redo her yard. Deb had a set amount of money to spend and could not provide for the removal of three large, unattractive boulders in the middle of the lawn. In a nonhypnotic example of utilization, the creative landscaper *incorporated* the boulders into his plan, and by adding certain trees, vines, and decorative stone he *transformed* the boulders into ornamental elements of the yard.

You may have heard the old maxim, "If life hands you lemons, make lemonade." This is also an example of utilization. Similarly, when a tennis player is the recipient of a challenging serve, the player *accepts* this obstacle or challenge and makes the necessary adjustments with his or her arms, legs, or feet in order to *hit the ball where it is served*.

The best practitioner of utilization that I (GG) ever observed was an aged *curandera*, a Mexican-American folk healer (Gafner & Duckett, 1992). People could go to her house day or night. There were no insurance forms to fill out, you seldom had to wait, and if you could not pay, that was okay. The setting was warm and embracing.

Starting from the individual's position, and making use of the shared language, culture and belief system, she effected seemingly miraculous symptom relief with herbs and rituals. The *curandera* believes that patients have the ability to heal *within themselves* and that her job is to instigate the healing process.

With utilization we *accept* clients, rather than challenging or rejecting them. Each thought, word, deed, or problem is seen as unique, a *possible resource* in the service of therapy. In the first meeting we take careful note of a client's activities, interests, strongly held beliefs, and choice of language. Utilization enhances the therapeutic relationship because the therapist expresses *interest* and *curiosity* about all aspects of the person. It presupposes that clients already possess the needed resources to live meaningful lives, and that the therapist's job is to assist in their discovery. This approach uses behaviors or beliefs that already exist, as opposed to trying to implement completely new behaviors or force the adoption of beliefs that are alien to the client. Many writers (Combs & Freedman, 1990; Lankton & Lankton, 1986) have applauded this legacy of Milton Erickson, which allows therapists to approach their clients flexibly, permissively, and respectfully.

In utilization, solutions are seen as being contained in the problem (Gilligan, 1987). Treating anxiety with psychotherapy, for example, the therapist *recognizes* and *respects* the symptom and its purpose or function and does not attempt to elminate it. Instead, she gives directives that modify the frequency, intensity, duration, timing, or location of the symptom. Once its pattern is altered, the symptom begins to dissipate (Lankton & Lankton, 1986).

In a hypnotic induction, the therapist recognizes, or paces, a client's sighs, blinking, or rigid beliefs, and then leads, or directs, the client in the desired direction (Gilligan, 1987). For example, we may say to the client, "Noticing a change in your breathing, or those eyes blinking, and recognizing strong convictions about things can be the first steps in developing an appreciation for going deeper and deeper into trance. . . ." The therapist can similarly utilize an intrusive noise, such as people talking in the hallway: " . . . and paying attention to many things, inside and outside, you may begin to notice how all of these things can lead you deeper and deeper into a pleasant state of relaxation. . . ."

Dr. Brent Geary of the Erickson Foundation once stated, "Everything can be utilized, and you won't utilize everything" (personal communication, 1998). This put utilization into focus for me (SB). We suggest that you start by taking the most salient aspect of the client's presentation—e.g., anger, dysphoria, rigidity, or narcissism—reframe it, and use it as a building block in your induction. Anger, for example, can be utilized accordingly: "Augie, someone one time sat there in that same chair and went deeply into trance, and I remember how that man, too, had an *appreciation for intensity of expression and strong feeling*, and it was natural for him to begin to notice unique and *special sensations* in his body, a warmth or heaviness in his feet, or was it a coldness or tingling in his hands, or some other interesting feeling someplace else?"

THE SETTING

A quiet, comfortable office is of inestimable assistance in hypnotherapy. In my office at the Tucson, Arizona, V.A., I (GG) have a large bulletin board covered with pictures, old sheet music, and similar material, and there are colorful Mexican ceramic parrots hanging from the ceiling. Consequently, there is a lot to choose from when clients are asked to experience eye fixation. It also helps to have a recliner for those who want to put their feet up, as well as a sturdy chair, not too low to the ground, for older clients or those with back pain.

In my office at the V.A. clinic in Mesa, Arizona, I (SB) have a framed poem entitled "Friend in the Mirror" by Edward Cunningham. This serves as a common focal point for eye fixation inductions. Occasional noise from the hallway or adjoining rooms must be contended with at both offices. I (SB) often make suggestions for clients to allow background noise to remain just outside their conscious awareness, or not to notice or respond to anything but the sound of my voice. We have also experimented with a variety of machines that produce background noises. There are many inexpensive solid state units that produce the sound of ocean waves, tropical rain, croaking frogs, and myriad other sounds. I (GG) have found that children often prefer the tick-tick sound of a metronome. Clients' sense of control is enhanced when they are allowed to choose a certain background sound or none at all. We have found that clients seem to prefer the ocean wave sound.

Be prepared for clients to take you at your word when you tell them to sit in any chair they want or to do anything else they need to do to feel comfortable. A few years ago Dr. Claire Frederick said in an American Society of Clinical Hypnosis (ASCH) workshop, "The good thing about hypnosis is that *anything is okay.*" She meant that the therapist should be permissive and accepting of any response elicited from the client. Her statement comes back to me (GG) when I think of interesting and unpredictable ways in which clients have responded. One woman chose to lay suggestively on the couch. A 400-pound man lay on his back on the floor and later had great difficulty getting to his feet. One man, who suffered from back pain and could not tolerate sitting, went into trance standing up. He soon fell asleep, started to rock back and forth, and had to be awakened before he fell over.

At the V.A. we see a number of hearing-impaired clients. Loud voices are not conducive to trancework, so we use an audio amplifier to bypass this problem. Also, at the conclusion of therapy we make clients a personalized audiotape that contains an induction, a deepening script, and a story that captures key elements of therapy. In our Stress Management Program at the Tucson V.A., clients are typically seen for six sessions or less. Some of these clients have generalized anxiety disorder and posttraumatic stress disorder. However, many present with a range of psychotic disorders. We administer a Beck Anxiety Inventory at the beginning and end of treatment. Clients are told that the purpose of treatment is "not to eliminate anxiety, but to just take the edge off of it; to give you some tools to keep it from getting out of hand."

Both long- and short-term clients respond very well to the inductions and deepenings in this book and often show an objective reduction in anxiety symptoms. They are grateful for a method that respects their own individual differences and helps utilize resources they have within themselves. Erickson is said to have told clients, "My voice will go with you" (Rosen, 1982). There are many ways your voice can go with your clients. Two techniques we use are the individualized audiotape and the installation of an anchor, or cue (e.g., one deep breath). Whether the goal is relaxation, ego-strengthening, pain management or some other application, these techniques help clients trigger whatever they experienced in their sessions. Some clients do not listen to their audiotape. Instead, they value it as a transitional object, a "security blanket" to assist them in maintaining their goal.

YOUR VOICE

Beginning practitioners of hypnotherapy usually have a number of questions about their voice. They find little comfort in answers along the lines of "with practice you will find your own voice." Therapists who have seen a videotape of Dr. Kay Thompson may try to mimic her. They might remember Milton Erickson from a vintage tape and attempt to reproduce his raspy, grandfatherly tone when he says, "Yes, tha-a-a-t's right. . . . "

Some effective hypnotherapists always speak in a low, boring monotone with little modulation. Others begin their hypnotic patter in a conversational voice and ever so gradually lower the volume and slow the tempo until they have reached their hypnotic voice. Others modulate their voice at different times during the induction or therapy portion, perhaps slowing down or lowering the volume to emphasize key suggestions.

We tell interns, "You have your conversational voice, your psychotherapy voice, and then you have your *hypnotic voice*." We recommend practice with a tape recorder, trying many different things, until they find a voice that is comfortable to them. Some have said, "But I don't like the sound of my voice," and we insist they find a voice that they like. We also have a story we tell interns—about a person who finds his voice.

HOW TO USE THIS BOOK

The practitioner new to hypnotherapy may wish to start at the beginning, where we illustrate relatively easy-to-apply conversational inductions along with key terms and concepts. The glossary is also helpful in identifying key terms and clarifying their usage. Experienced clinicians can also benefit from some of the inductions in Chapter 2, which may bolster their repertoire. However, those who are comfortable with stock inductions may wish to jump ahead to the following chapters, where more elaborate inductions are demonstrated.

Many older practitioners rely exclusively on directive, authoritarian techniques such as those demonstrated in Chapter 5. Araoz (1988) is among those who draw a strong distinction between this "old hypnosis" and the "new hypnosis" in which many people have been trained in the past 30 years. The "old hypnosis" relied on standardized hypnotizability tests and highly directive techniques. In this school the client is instructed, for example, "Follow my hand with your eyes as I move it from your face up over your head, and as your eyes roll back, YOU WILL go deeply into trance"; or they might be told, once in trance, "You WILL be strong" or "You WILL lose weight."

Even methods akin to hypnosis, such as guided imagery, often employ rather authoritarian techniques. For example, "I want you to imagine that you are in a boat on a lake on a clear, sunny day. . . ." This presumes that such a setting is relaxing to the client, but being out on a lake might be terrifying to a client with a fear of deep water. This illustrates the importance of tailoring the approach to the client. In the U.S. alone there are dozens if not hundreds of programs where anyone can learn "to be a hypnotist." Many of these have minimal or no education or training requirements. These entities also espouse such one-size-fits-all techniques. Such approaches may foster exaggerated therapist confidence and could lead to negative consequences for both clients and professionals. This is why we underscore the need for requirements in education, training, and supervision in the practice of hypnotherapy.

For hundreds of years, hypnosis was done in an authoritarian manner, and some clients may still benefit from this approach. However, many clients today expect, and certainly are thought to benefit more from, a respectful, indirect, metaphorical approach that is geared to their particular orientations and interests. For the most part, clients who express an interest in trancework will be hypnotizable to some extent, and much clinical work can be done when a client is in a mild or medium trance. Milton Erickson and his successors (Erickson, Rossi, & Rossi, 1976; Gilligan, 1987; Haley, 1973; Lankton & Lankton, 1986; O'Hanlon, 1987) have popularized the more general and permissive approach that is the "new hypnosis." Most of the inductions in this book adhere to this philosophy.

In our training program at the Tucson V.A., we expect trainees to achieve competency in at least four inductions. (Internships in different disciplines vary from nine months to a year.) Following practice reading conversational or embedded-meaning inductions in their respective hypnosis training group, interns usually continue reading inductions in their work with clients, who respond well to these inductions. Eventually, they progress to more elaborate inductions, and by the time they are done they can successfully ad lib inductions.

Hypnotherapists should keep in mind the law of parsimony. In hypnotic inductions, less is more, so the simplest key should be used that opens the door. In some cases, the door is already halfway open and all that is needed are inductions such as those in Chapter 2. Other times the door is actually wide open. For example, some experienced clients only need to be asked to sit back and go into trance. For other clients, especially those with unconscious resistance, you may need to try various keys before the door will open. The inductions in Chapters 3 and 4 will be very useful for these clients.

Throughout this book we have tried to illustrate some of the wide array of both inductions and deepenings. We encourage you to experiment with these, take something from one and something from another, to see what works for you and your clients. We never know what will work with a particular client until we *try something—* an induction or therapeutic application—and then, based on client response, we keep fine-tuning and individualizing the approach. Similarly, you will not know what you are personally comfortable with, and what you can place your confidence in, until you try different inductions. Tailoring hypnotherapy to the individual client is important, but equally consequential to us is the *development of the therapist*. We attend workshops and training on hypnosis, but we also regularly collaborate with our peers, exchanging therapeutic stories and consulting with each other via e-mail, seeking input on applications for various clinical problems.

Most of all, we hope that the inductions in this book will stimulate your own creativity, resourcefulness, and learning, allowing you to continually improve your hypnotherapy skills.

2

General Conversational Inductions

For all the inductions in this book, clients are asked to choose a comfortable place and settle into a comfortable position. They are told that, at any time, they can move around, adjust their position, speak aloud, or do anything else that will allow their comfort to deepen. They are asked to do a mental scan of their body in order to locate any discomfort. If they report tension in their neck, for example, the therapist makes note of this index feeling.

EYE FIXATION

We devised this induction for a research protocol involving hypnosis and chronic PTSD at the Tucson V.A. Many clients with PTSD do not wish to close their eyes. Accordingly, this induction allows for either eye fixation or eye closure. We eventually adopted this induction as an all-purpose one for many clients. Notice that the induction contains many suggestions for feelings in the body. The greater the clients' *experience* of trance—especially ideosensory feeling, time distortion, and dissociation—the more they will believe in it (Hammond, 1994). It is important to ratify these phenomena at the end of the session, especially the first time.

Induction

With your eyes, I would like you to select a spot on the wall, or the ceiling, or *anywhere you like*, and focus on that spot, and when you have done so, let me know by nodding your head . . . *that's the way*.

permissive suggestion

pacing

Now, as you're looking at that spot, (client's name), you may begin to notice a *fuzziness* or *haziness* in that spot out there. Some people find that that spot out there begins to change in *shape*, or *size*, or *color*, maybe getting *bigger*, or *smaller*, or *staying just the same*, and you will find that your eyes have a tendency to blink, *and* your eyes *may gently close*, all by themselves . . . or some people find that they are more comfortable *continuing to look at that spot*, which is just fine. Sometimes a kind of tunnel vision can develop when a person looks at any one spot for a length of time, *and* a person can become especially absorbed in that spot way out there.

suggestion covering all possibilities

linking word

permissive suggestion

linking word

Perhaps you've already begun to notice your breathing, (client's name), *how your rate of breathing has started to change*, maybe almost imperceptibly, and *as you breathe in* comfort and relaxation, *you can begin* to *slow down* your mind, and *slow down* your body with each comfortable breath in; *and any nervousness or tension, you can*

implication

contingent suggestion repetition

blow that out each time you exhale.
That's the way . . . , absolutely *nothing
at all to do or know or change or even
think about*, and it can be very com-
forting to know that all you really have
to do is just sit there and breathe,
always being in the *driver's seat*, ever so
gradually beginning to *slow down* both
your mind and your body.

contingent suggestion
(continued)
not knowing/not doing

metaphor
repetition

    Everyone, (client's name), *has experi-
enced relaxation*, perhaps the *warm* sun
on your skin on a *cold* day . . . or a
refreshing breeze blowing against your
face on a hot day . . . or other times *like
driving a car*, or *listening to pleasant
music, or something else* that comes to
mind . . . where you become more and
more absorbed in a satisfying experience, when time might seem to *speed
up*, or *slow down*, when a *minute can
seem like an hour, or an hour like a
minute*, or maybe it's simply a matter of
losing track of time.

truism

apposition of opposites

*naturalistic trance
experiences*

apposition of opposites

*bind of comparable
alternatives*

    Now, (client's name), *getting up this
morning, coming over here today like
you did, (sunny/cloudy/warm) day that
it is outside, waiting for a while in the
waiting room, then walking down that
hall and coming in here, and sitting
down there*, I know that *you can begin
to experience a very enjoyable sense of
relaxation*. I can't know if, with the
front part of your mind, you wondered
about going lightly and swiftly into a
moderate state of relaxation, or instead, with the *back part of your mind*,
you imagined going more slowly and
profoundly into a deeper state of
trance, which can be like an *entrance*

truisms

suggestion

*conscious/unconscious
double bind*

into another state, but it really doesn't matter because whatever happens is okay, as the experience is yours and yours alone, private and internal, something for you to enjoy and appreciate.

Now (client's name), while I'm talking to you today, you will hear an occasional *pause* . . . or *silence* . . . times when there are no words, and those can be times to let your experience deepen . . . a *pause* . . . or a *silence* . . . and you may hear every word I say, or the words might drift in, and drift out. At the same time, you will begin to notice feelings that invariably happen in your body . . . perhaps a *tingling or numbness* in one hand, or both hands, or maybe a *coolness or warmth,* or *heaviness or lightness, or some other curious feeling.* These feelings or sensations usually happen in a person's extremities, but they may occur somewhere else in your body, *effortlessly, all by themselves, without any conscious attempt on your part,* or simply as a part of letting go just a bit at a time. *One person* one time said (s)he could detect a definite heaviness in (her) his feet and (s)he could hardly move *those* feet, almost like (s)he was wearing very heavy Western boots. *Another person* commented that (her) his hands felt *detached* from the rest of (her) him while at the same time (s)he was very aware of (her) his toes as (s)he curled them up inside (her) his shoes. *One (wo)man* reported that (s)he noticed an interesting prickliness in (her) his

pun/embedded meaning

seeding

seeding (activated)

suggestion covering all possibilities

involuntariness

metaphor

dissociation

metaphor

dissociation

metaphor

scalp, along with a dryness in (her) his mouth. I remember *one person* who was intrigued by an itchiness in (her) his right ear lobe, strange as that might seem. Whatever feelings you begin to notice, they are your experience, and yours alone, all part of becoming more and more *deeply and comfortably relaxed* . . . (pause) . . . Noticing those feelings, you can begin to appreciate, really appreciate and enjoy, both your body and your mind *slowing down, deeper and deeper,* into a very *comfortable state of relaxation* . . . (pause) . . . .

Many people find it *interesting*, maybe even *curious*, how they can pay attention to what's going on inside— feelings, thoughts, and sensations— and also focus on what's going on outside at the same time. On the outside— the feeling of thc chair beneath you, *those* hands out there, and the words— after all it's *your ears I'm speaking to* . . . at the same time it's also common, to have *part of you noticing the process*, noticing you going into trance, just wondering about it all. We call this "the hidden observer," and it's rather interesting how all these things can be going on at the same time, and all the while you can be *in the driver's seat*. One person one time called this *controlling letting go*, while another called it *letting go of control*, and I still get confused by the two of them.

Everybody's mind has a front part and a back part, the front part that pays attention to your breathing, and the words, and the feelings developing

metaphor

repetition
seeding (activated)

repetition

seeding (activated)

hypnotic language

dissociation
dissociation

hidden observer

metaphor

bind of comparable alternatives

in your body; and the *back of the mind*, the part that is like the *big part of an iceberg* . . . you don't see it, but you know it's there, underneath the water, watchful, waiting, cautious, private . . . deep inside . . . inside there where you have your imagination, and intuition, the part of your mind that can help you now when you need it the most. . . .

unconscious process

That's the way, (client's name), breathing comfortably, more and more deeply relaxed, *nothing consciously to do or know or think about*, letting it happen all by itself.

not knowing/not doing

Now (client's name), before starting out down the road, it can be very comfortable to open the door, and then sit there behind the wheel, *being the one who drives*. . . . Once out on the road, a person *speeds up*, and then *slows down*. *Speeding up*, and other times *slowing down*. More and more deeply and comfortably relaxed, breathing in, and breathing out.

metaphor

apposition of opposites

suggestion

Deepening

Now, in a moment, (client's name), I'm going to count backward, down from ten to one, and as those numbers go backward, down from ten to one, I'd like you to *imagine*, just *imagine*, yourself sinking a bit deeper and deeper into an even more comfortable and satisfying state of relaxation, as I begin to count now, ten, nine, ... (Client's name), when you are sufficiently deep in order to do the work you need to do today, you can let me know by nodding your head . . . very good.

REALERTING

Following the therapy portion of trancework, the client is realerted. We often say something like this in a voice that is higher in volume:

"In a moment I'm going to count from one up to five and by the time my voice gets up to three, or four, or five, you can then resume your normal waking state. One . . . two . . ."

DEBRIEFING

Several minutes should be spent debriefing the client, especially in the first few sessions of trancework. The client may share important basic information, e.g., "You need to speak louder," or let you know that something you said was distracting. The overall goal for the first session is for the client to feel comfortable. Whatever you can do or say to aid in the client's comfort will facilitate the therapy process. This may be as simple as making the room darker or something more involved like choosing a different kind of induction. Asking for feedback provides the information you need to individualize and fine-tune your approach with a particular client.

Another important aspect of debriefing involves eliciting and ratifying (reinforcing) trance phenomena. You may ask open-ended questions such as "How do you feel?" or "How does your body feel?" or, more specifically, "How does your left hand feel? And your right?" Time distortion is detected with a question such as "Without looking at the clock, what time would you guess it is right now?" Also, clients are queried regarding the index feeling. If they report a feeling of relief, e.g., "My neck doesn't feel so tight," this also ratifies trance.

NOTES FOR PRACTICE

You may notice that the client's name is mentioned frequently. Even in a deep level of trance (and, in fact, in the delta stage of sleep) people *hear* their name, so you are connecting with them in a strong and personal way. Repetition is also used for important suggestions. A general rule is: If it is important, repeat it, either the same way or in different ways, perhaps buttressing the idea with metaphor. You may notice that in the deepening the person is asked to *imagine* going deeper. In a more authoritarian induction clients would be asked *to do* something in their mind, for example, walk down a staircase. It is difficult for a client to resist simply imagining something.

In deepening, the client is asked for a head nod to verify subjective depth. What if you receive no head nod? Maybe you did not wait long enough. Always give clients at least a minute to respond. Sometimes when questioned during debriefing, they say, "Oh, I thought I did nod my head." At any rate, if you don't get a discernible response, just move on.

We make careful note of everything clients tell us after being re-alerted, especially during the first few sessions. If they report a pleasant warmth in their chest, in the next session we may say, "I wonder when you will begin to notice that pleasant feeling beginning to develop in your chest. . . ." If they say something was negative or distracting, like a noise in the hall, next session we may say, ". . . and all the sounds you hear can be incorporated into your experience as you notice yourself going deeper and deeper . . ." In these ways, we utilize the client's experience in the service of therapy.

DON'T TRY TOO HARD

This induction may be the hypnotic equivalent of the progressive muscle relaxation (PMR) technique. Clients are not asked to tense and relax their muscles as in PMR; however, in this induction you directly suggest relaxation in successive parts of the body. More concrete, bodily-oriented individuals, as well as adolescents and children, may respond favorably to this induction, which is more authoritarian than the previous one. Notice that the suggestion for eye closure is rather firm and directive, not permissive and general like the previous induction, which allowed for either continued eye fixation or eye closure. Accordingly, you need to be prepared to pace the client's response in case eye closure does not occur, for example, ". . . or your eyes may find it more comfortable to remain open as your body continues to become more relaxed with each deep breath. . . ."

Communicating or "dancing" with the client requires that you periodically look up from the script and monitor the client's response. With practice and experience, you will not have to rely on a prepared script, and monitoring, pacing, and leading will become much easier.

As these scripts are written to be read aloud (and to have a hypnotic effect), conventional rules for writing are not followed. Sentences that begin with "and," incomplete and run-on sentences, and even double or triple negatives are included purposely.

The concept of unconscious mind is seeded in pre-trance discussion. The therapist may tell the client that the unconscious mind is like the big part of the iceberg, largely unseen beneath the water, or perhaps the therapist wonders aloud, "I wonder how your unconscious mind will benefit from this experience today. . . ."

Induction

(Client's name), *don't try too hard to make things happen, and don't try to stop things from happening.* Just allow your *imagination* to wander as you notice things going on, perhaps *interesting* or *curious* thoughts or sensations, maybe on the *inside* or the *outside, or both at the same* time. *You don't have to think, or reply, or try to do anything at all.* In fact, it *isn't even necessary to listen* carefully to what I'm saying because your *unconscious mind will inevitably pay attention* to anything important, without any conscious effort on your part. Now, (client's name), perhaps you *thought ahead of time* about this experience today. Maybe it *crossed your mind yesterday or the day before, or maybe you wondered about it today* or in the waiting room a few minutes ago, and perhaps right now *a part of you is observing the process while the rest of you just goes along with the experience,* which is just fine, because beginning now you can *let yourself go* into just as light or deep a trance as you would like.

As you hear my voice you can allow your body to relax as deeply as you can. Now take several deep breaths, just as deep as you'd like . . . very good, that's the way. . . . A deep breath can feel so very comfortable and satisfying.

bind of comparable alternatives

hypnotic language

bind of comparable alternatives
not knowing / not doing

restraint

suggestion

truisms

hidden observer

suggestion

contingent suggestion

(If client's eyes are not already closed) You may begin to notice that your *eyes*, and particularly your *eyelids*, may feel very, very *drowsy, heavy and somewhat sleepy . . . and* as they begin to blink, they may become especially *tired and heavy*, and *when* it is hard to keep them open, *those* eyes may wish to close *all by themselves*, that's the way . . . changing perspective . . . and going inside can be a most *curious* contrast.

suggestion

linking word
suggestion
implication
dissociation
involuntariness

hypnotic language

The feeling that you can attain in your body is a sensation of *complete and total muscular relaxation . . .* just relaxing into a deep and very *relaxed state . . .* simply listening to my voice . . . and *drifting* into a very, very pleasant state of mind . . . a body that is *free from all tension and tightness, free from stress and strain.* As you listen to my voice guiding you into a total and *complete state of relaxation . . .* your mind, your body . . . the muscular system, the nervous system . . . *limp, relaxed* muscles . . . and your *breathing* is the essence of deep, *deep relaxation.* Your entire body is becoming *completely and totally relaxed*, your *head . . . your face . . . your neck . . . shoulders . . . back . . . chest . . . arms . . . completely relaxed*, very deeply relaxed, your *mind* and your *body*, relaxed, at ease, free from tension, tightness, stress and strain.

repetition

repetition

suggestion

repetition

suggestion

Feeling *secure and at rest.* Enjoying the sense of *quietness* and calmness. No pressure, no need to rush, no one to please, no one to satisfy. This is just *your* time to *rest and enjoy* a gentle

suggestion

peacefulness. Just letting go, quietly and gently, with nothing to bother you, and nothing to disturb you.

While you *sit there* quietly, you can *notice your breathing*, and at the same time you *recognize* you are moving deeper and deeper into relaxation. That's the way. . . .

contingent suggestion

As soon as your unconscious mind is ready to move deeper into trance, you can raise your right index finger. Good. You know, I once knew *a woman* who let her unconscious mind identify issues that had been bothering her. As she let her unconscious mind look *into* the solutions, that were already there *in*side her, she began to feel more and more at ease. And as you allow your own imag*in*ation to wander, peering into your own inside issues, *your conscious mind may think about solutions, while your unconscious mind considers their implications; or perhaps your unconscious mind will generate some solutions, while your conscious mind wonders what the result might be*

metaphor

embedded meaning/ suggestion for internal search

conscious-unconscious double bind

And now, *letting that comfort* and calmness flow, out to every part of you. Bringing such a sense of *peacefulness, and quiet, and calm*, that any inner stresses can also relax. Allowing all the stress and strain to *just fade into the background*, and become more and more distant, farther and farther away . . . .

suggestion

And now I'm going to give you some quiet time, to continue experiencing a deep level of relaxation, enjoying it in your own way. (Allow about 90 seconds.)

Deepening

(Client's name), I would like you to imagine, just imagine in your mind, a staircase, an elevator, or an escalator, something that goes down one floor at a time. When you have one of those in your mind, let me know by nodding your head. . . . Good, that's the way.

Now I'd like you to go down that staircase or whatever you're picturing in your mind, down from ten to one, at your own pace, in your own way, letting your experience deepen with each number down, and when you've gotten there, you will know and I will know because you will take one more deep, comfortable breath. . . . Good, that's the way.

REALERTING

After therapy, the client may be realerted with the following: "In a few moments, your eyes will open. When you awaken, you may *forget to remember*, or you *may remember to forget* (bind of comparable alternatives/suggestion for amnesia) the important unconscious work you did here today. Soon, but not just yet, you'll be opening your eyes. You will feel great, just as though you have had a very pleasant nap. Your whole body will feel relaxed and refreshed. Everything about you will be comfortable and relaxed, your body and your mind, very relaxed and comfortable. And now, take several refreshing, energizing breaths and let yourself become fully alert and awake."

DEBRIEFING

As this induction is heavily oriented toward bodily relaxation, trance-ratifying questions should be directed accordingly. Since a suggestion for amnesia was given at the end, you may ask, "Do you have any conscious recollection of unconscious things that came to mind back there when you raised your finger?"

NOTES FOR PRACTICE

A period of silence is provided at the end of the induction. A "quiet time" such as this is one of the most effective deepening techniques we know, and it certainly follows the law of parsimony: less is more, and sometimes the *absence* of our words can be highly beneficial. For many clients, further deepening will be unnecessary.

The formal deepening portion is very permissive and, in effect, allows for clients to go down *any way* they choose. This is important for people with pain or without mobility.

Notice that nothing is taken for granted. You know when they are ready to go deeper because they respond with a finger signal. When you ask the person to imagine something, you verify it by eliciting a head nod or some other signal. Occasionally they may not signal. If that happens, some therapists repeat the request. However, we believe that this may create a power struggle or possibly lead clients to think that they have failed or "got it wrong." Such negative situations are probably best avoided by simply moving on if no response is forthcoming. You can broach the problem during debriefing.

This induction introduced another way for the client to communicate in trance: the finger signal. To be effective, clients must place their hands on their lap where you can see them. What if you ask for a finger signal with the right hand and they move their *left* index finger? It may mean the client is trying her best to cooperate. If confounding responses continue in subsequent sessions, it may be better to use a head nod instead. Finger signals will be discussed further with other inductions.

It is normal for clients to forget some or all of what you tell them during trancework. However, you may nurture this process with suggestions for amnesia, as in this induction. Erickson and others believed that most problem-solving occurs at the level of the unconscious. Amnesia allows unconscious work to continue without interference from the conscious mind. Other ways to facilitate amnesia will be addressed in subsequent inductions.

CREATING OR RE-EXPERIENCING A PLEASANT SCENE

This induction, like the Perceiving Sensations induction (p. 31), is very economical. It may appear to be quite simple, which it is, but that should not imply that it is easy. Clinicians who can use these inductions effectively usually have some previous hypnotherapy experience and already know some other inductions. People trained in neurolinguistic programming (Bandler & Grinder, 1982) as well as hypnosis often prefer these inductions because they utilize the client's current, ongoing behavior. These are also the inductions of choice among many Ericksonian hypnotherapists in Mexico (Perez,

1994; Robles, 1993), where the rich culture and language may aid in joining with a person's sensory experience.

Compared to conventional psychotherapy, hypnotherapy accelerates rapport because clients must feel trust if the therapist is to lead them through the steps of trancework. Trust and rapport are expedited even more with inductions such as this one, in which the therapist closely observes clients, pacing and leading their behavior. The therapist's leverage for influencing behavioral change may also be accelerated in very "personal" inductions such as these, in which client and therapist seem to dance in sync.

We have found that clients who do not close their eyes have difficulty experiencing these inductions. Accordingly, we like to find out about eye closure before we begin. We may say, for example, "Do this for me, please: Close your eyes for a second or two . . . good . . . now go ahead and close your eyes while I count to ten . . . good, how did that feel?" We then ask if they would like to keep their eyes closed throughout today's trancework in order to have a more complete and *pleasant* (seeding) experience. Most people will say yes, but if the answer is no, we usually go to another induction, such as Eye Fixation or Don't Try Too Hard. If people feel uncomfortable with eye closure, this must be respected.

Induction

As you sit back and begin to feel comfortably relaxed, I would like you to let those eyes gently close . . . that's the way . . . recognizing that *with those eyes closed you can go inside* very *pleasantly*, accessing memories, past experiences, or other meaningful events, times gone by when you felt good. Now, (client's name), I'd like you to take two deep, refreshing breaths *and as you release that second breath you can drift* even more deeply into a satisfying a *pleasant* state of relaxation. . . . Now, (client's name), a few seconds ago when I mentioned thinking about a	*contingent suggestion* *implication* *seeding* (activated) *linking word* *implication* *seeding* (activated)

pleasant time from the past, perhaps   *seeding* (activated)
something came to mind, and if so, you
may nod your head . . . (if a head nod is
not forthcoming) and, if not, *you can*   *permissive suggestion*
retrieve or even just imagine experienc-
ing something *pleasant* now, anything   *seeding* (activated)
you like. . . . You don't have to say what
it is and you can just enjoy it internally
and privately . . . (if a head nod still has
not happened), and it can be anything
you like, anything at all. One time *a*   *metaphor*
person sitting right there thought about
a nice *warm bath*, and another thought
about a *cool shower*, a walk in the   *apposition of opposites*
woods or along the beach, and *when*
you have that pleasant experience there,   *implication*
you may nod your head . . . good . . .
breathing comfortably and relaxed,
just letting it happen all by itself.

   Now, (client's name), in your mind
there, I'd like you to notice if you're   *dissociative language*
inside or *outside* . . . if it's *daytime* or
nighttime, and perhaps you even know
approximately what time it is . . . *hours*   *apposition of opposites*
and *minutes*, clock time, which isn't
like trance time . . . and if it's *light* or
dark . . . just noticing things *inside* as
well as *outside* . . .

   Just *feel* the temperature on your   *suggestions*
skin . . . and *notice* all the other things
around you and *notice* colors around
you . . . and patterns . . . and sounds . . .
or silence.

   Feel each part of your body and the
movements, there in that place, . . . and
notice your breathing . . . the clothes
you are wearing . . . their texture on
your skin . . . on your arms or perhaps
your back . . . or maybe somewhere else,

and *feel* your breath . . . there where you
are in that pleasant place, *enjoying* and
appreciating it. . . .

Deepening

(Client's name), among all the different aspects of your pleasant
experience, perhaps there is one very vivid or memorable thing,
maybe a feeling on your skin, maybe the thought of being there in that
experience, maybe a color or a scent, a deep breath, or something
else. Now in a moment I'm going to ask you to imagine one of those
things, that's the way, and when one very pleasant thing from that
experience comes to mind, let me know by nodding your head . . .
good . . . and I'd like you to continue thinking of that one thing now,
feeling and experiencing it, while I count out loud, from ten down to
one, and as those numbers descend you can imagine yourself sinking even deeper into that pleasant experience . . . ten . . . nine . . . .

Realerting

After the therapy portion, the client may be realerted (speaking with
a bit more volume) by, "As I count from one up to five you will begin
to feel alert, and by the time my voice gets up to five you will feel
alert and refreshed . . . one . . . two . . . ."

Debriefing

Clients are often fascinated by the way they can become absorbed in
a rather simple exercise, especially one that is generated from their
own experience. You might ask, "Do you wish to tell me what pleasant situation you imagined?" Most clients will be eager to reveal this.
Then foster their interest or fascination by asking about the quality
of their experience, e.g., "Tell me more about walking along that
beach. . . ." It is important to focus on the aspect of the imaginal
experience elicited in the deepening, as this will both ratify trance
and give you valuable information about the client's capacity for
imaginal absorption.

Notes for Practice

This induction works best if drawn out with ample pauses and
silences, which allow the client time to experience suggestions.

Notice how *pleasant* was seeded early on, and later activated, in the induction.

Occasionally, clients may be unable to imagine something when asked to do so. If you do not receive a head nod, simply proceed with something like, "I'm going to count down now from ten to one and as those numbers descend you can imagine, in your own way, going deeper and deeper into trance." Debriefing is vital in finding out what does work and what does not work for the client. With this information, you can adapt subsequent trancework to the client's particular needs. We take note of virtually everything the client says during debriefing, as these responses are most valuable in utilization. Fragments, curious impressions, or idle wonderings can become building blocks of therapy. The essence of utilization is being able to convert or reframe something negative ("If life hands you lemons, make lemonade"). For example, if a client reports, "All I could think about was my dry mouth and how I didn't swallow," then next session we would add, " . . . and some people find it most curious—almost to the point of distraction—how they can notice certain feelings and sensations in their body, maybe something rather different than they expected, and these responses are perfectly normal and natural, and in fact sometimes people can become absorbed in these things, deepening their experience, and other times people pay passing notice before turning to something else in their body that catches their attention. . . ."

In this induction you need to be ready to pace and lead a range of behaviors that may arise: changes in breathing, moving around in the chair, flushing of the cheeks, eye flutter, etc. Eye flutter may mean distress or incongruence (feeling as if something doesn't "fit"). The client may not remember this fleeting moment when queried during debriefing, so it is advisable to make a mental note of what you are saying when eye flutter occurs.

It is easy to understand how some clients think you can actually read their minds when you become adept at pacing and leading. For example, the client experiences eye flutter, which is followed by a positional shift and a long sigh. Your response is " . . . and sometimes in trance a person may experience something upsetting, or maybe a strange thought or feeling, which can lead to changing position—or even perspective—and exhaling deeply can help a person appreciate the comfort of trance on an even deeper level. . . ."

PERCEIVING SENSATIONS

Like the Creating or Re-experiencing a Pleasant Scene induction, clients find this induction very personal, eliciting the experience of the therapist "dancing" with them. As in the previous induction, you need to be prepared to pace and lead a variety of possible nonverbal behaviors.

Pre-trance discussion is used to seed *outside* and *inside*, which is central to the experience of this induction. We may ask clients, "What's the weather like *outside* right now?" or, "The temperature in here, *inside* this room, how does it feel to you?" Even more directly, we may tell them, "Today in the induction I'm going to ask you to experience some things *inside* and *outside*. Many people find this a very interesting experience, something in which they can become very absorbed." Clients are also prepared for eye closure: "In a moment I'm going to ask you to look around the room and notice some things, and then ask you to close your eyes so we can draw a contrast between the two experiences. How does that sound?" If they decline, we tell them that is fine and simply proceed with something else.

Induction

(Client's name), *notice* the different colors and patterns *out* there, *in* this room, how one thing is very different from something else . . . shapes . . . sizes . . . colors . . . patterns . . . that's the way,	*suggestion* *apposition of opposites*
and after noticing those things *you may find it interesting to close your eyes and contrast* in your mind what you re-member of those colors . . . shapes . . . sizes, and everything else.	*linking word* *implication*
(If the client's eyes have closed) Through your eyelids you can feel, just sense, the *brightness* or *darkness* of this room . . . and with your ears you can listen to the sounds . . . and the sound of my voice . . . and notice how each sound, instead of being a distraction,	*apposition of opposites*

can help you to be more in touch with   implication
yourself as you begin to go inside . . . *and*
there's nothing whatsoever that you have
to consciously do or know or think about,   not knowing/not doing
as you go more and more inside. . . .

You can feel your weight supported
by that chair . . . and your feet on the   truisms
ground. Maybe *you can feel* those
things lightly or intensely . . . and there's
the texture of the chair . . . and maybe
your *right* foot *down* there feels one   apposition of opposites
way, different from your *left* hand *up*
there, or your *left* foot on the floor per-
ceives the inside of your shoe in a way
that is different from what your *right*
hand detects up above. Just noticing
many things, that's the way. . . .

The shirt (dress, top, etc.) touching
your arm, either the right or the left,
there are places the *fabric touches* . . .
and others where it does not . . . and
perhaps the *collar* of that garment *feels*   truisms
smoother, or rougher, up there than it
does where it *touches your chest,* or
your back . . . just noticing this and
many other things . . . on one foot, *feel-*
ing your heel in your shoe, or your toes,
the *left* side versus the *right* side, *top*   apposition of opposites
of the foot, *bottom* of the foot. . . . *One*
person one time found herself curling   metaphor
up her toes each time she inhaled, and
I can't remember if one or both of those   amnesia
things allowed her to go deeper and
deeper into trance.

Another person took great care to   metaphor
notice the contrasting feeling of the
ring on one hand with the feeling of his
watch on the other wrist. By *noticing*   suggestion
these things he invariably became

more and more *absorbed* in the total
experience, things outside . . . and espe-
cially *inside* because *going inside* is   *seed* (activated)
invariably most curious and interest-
ing. . . .

(pause for several seconds)

Deepening

I'm going to count down now from ten to one, and as I count backward I'm going to tell you a little story called "The Three Lessons."
As those numbers go down, I'd like you to imagine yourself sinking
deeper and deeper into an even more comfortable and pleasant state
of relaxation.

Ten . . . nine . . . Once, not too long ago, there was a young girl who
lived in another state. I don't remember if it was in Washington or
Georgia or someplace else. Eight . . . seven . . . She heard about a wise
elderly woman who lived deep in the woods, and she figured that the
wise woman was someone who could help her with her problem, so
she went to a lot of trouble to find directions to her house, and once
she did, she set out through the forest. Six . . . five . . . It was late
November and it was cold. She could see her breath, and as she
passed an icy stream she bent down and put her hand into the cold,
cold water. Eventually, up ahead in a clearing, she saw the house,
and when she got there she knocked on the door. From inside she
heard a voice that said, "You may come in," which was lesson number one. Four . . . three . . . It was warm in the house and she looked
around at all the things in there . . . and finally she could contain herself no longer and blurted out, "I want to know everything you know
so I can help myself with my problem," and the wise woman looked
deeply into the girl's eyes and said, "I see that you already know
everything that you need to know except that you don't yet know that
you already know all those things," which was lesson number two.

Finally, as it was nearing the time to go, the young girl didn't know
if a minute had passed or an hour. She looked up again at the wise
woman who said, "You must listen very closely," which was lesson
number three. The young woman left and we know that everything
worked out just fine for her . . . two . . . and one . . .

REALERTING

The client may be realerted by counting from one to five as in the previous induction. You may also try a more general and permissive realerting such as, "Taking as much time as you need, let yourself reawaken, and when you're ready, you may open your eyes."

DEBRIEFING

General questions that address feelings, sensations, thoughts and perceptions in the induction will provide you with valuable information for future trancework. For example, a client may state, "I really went deeper when I felt the chair supporting my body" or, negatively, "I came out of trance for a while when you mentioned the ring on my finger because it reminded me of my divorce." In that case, you should avoid mentioning rings in the future. As for experiencing her body sinking into the chair, next time you may be able to induce trance with something as simple as, "Now, (client's name), I'd like you to fully experience your body supported by that chair, just sinking deeper and deeper into relaxation, taking as much time as you need, and when you feel sufficiently deep, you may signal with one deep, refreshing breath."

This deepening uses interspersal of a story with counting down. It can be seen as a "double deepening," because the client becomes absorbed in the story while simultaneously responding to a direct suggestion for deepening. We like to ask, "How do your hands feel?" Often clients will mention numbing or tingling in one hand, which may or may not be the hand that the young girl immersed in the cold stream. More than once we have heard clients say, "In my mind I saw the young girl (or man) put her right hand in the stream, but right now it's my *left* hand that feels numb—why is that?" We may answer such a question with, "Isn't it interesting what can happen when you let the unconscious mind take over?" In subsequent sessions we may capitalize on this with a statement such as, " . . . And beginning now you can let that numbness start to develop in your right hand . . . " or more permissively, " . . . I wonder which hand this time will begin to develop a numbness, a tingling, or some other curious sensation. . . . "

Stimulation of such wonderment and instigation of the client's *experiencing* such hypnotic phenomena go a long way toward ratifying trance, which is a strong ally of the therapeutic process.

NOTES FOR PRACTICE

Prior to beginning this induction, it is helpful for you to take careful note of jewelry, clothing, etc., so that these things can be accurately mentioned in the induction. Regarding a permissive rather than a directive realerting, be prepared for clients to take you at your word. Directing a client to "take as much time as you need" may result in his eyes being closed for much longer than you intended. After all, why should he interrupt a very pleasant experience? If another gentle reminder does not realert the client, I (GG) usually begin to work at my desk or undertake a similar activity until he eventually comes around.

You may notice that "The Three Lessons" story is adapted from Lee Wallas's (1985) story of the same name. We use this story often, even in standard talk therapy, because it accurately frames the role of therapist and client. Furthermore, its meta-message is potent and relevant: Clients have the needed resources within themselves.

The client's unconscious mind may accept or reject this metaphor, which we usually introduce early in hypnotherapy regardless of the induction used. More often than not, clients find it respectful of their own particular talents and abilities. Other times we wait for clients to provide their own metaphors. They may say something specific like "I want the world lifted from my shoulders," or make a more vague comparison, such as referring to life as a journey. We can then incorporate these into the induction, deepening, or therapy.

Metaphor combines the abstract and concrete in a way that enables people to go from the known and the sensed to the unknown and the symbolic. Siegelman (1990) sees a paradox here: The abstract is achieved through the concrete, i.e., through the senses, and most often through the visual mode. Metaphor's utility for therapists lies in its capacity to bridge the gap between the tangible and the ineffable. Its vividness connects to the world of felt and sensed experience. Accordingly, through the use of metaphor, we are more likely to *emotionally connect* with the client. Years after the conclusion of therapy, a client may mention, "You know, every once in a while I still dream about that old woman in the woods."

EARLY LEARNING SET

Milton Erickson was known to begin a conversational induction by casually taking an item such as a pen or coffee cup from his desk and simply talking about it, meandering from one thought to another, thereby inducing trance through a long monologue. Sometimes he would weave thoughts and memories about his own life into this hypnotic patter, and frequently he would include anecdotes about his children when they were young. Erickson would then shift the focus to the client's own early recollections, such as learning to walk, beginning school, and similar naturalistic experiences.

Focusing attention on early experiences is typical of Ericksonian utilization in that it employs universal experiences for the purpose of attentional absorption and then builds on these common behaviors. This approach is useful even for clients who have few memories of childhood. Many of these people have either raised children or been around them and these experiences can be similarly utilized.

The following induction is intentionally broader in scope than many early learning set inductions attempting to capture possible experiences—real or imagined—from both childhood and adolescence. We have found that "casting a wider net" affords clients more opportunity for self-referencing than inductions that concentrate only on the earliest years of development.

In pre-trance discussion we like to seed concepts such as *learn* or *remember*. This may be done metaphorically by referring to yourself, for example, "I *learned* long ago that comfort in trance is of paramount importance, so you may wish to sit back and close your eyes, or do anything else that helps you feel comfortable," or by using another person, "One day, another woman came in here, sat right down there in that same chair, and quite rapidly *learned* that she could *remember* many things that she had not thought about for years. . . ." We have found that clients often respond better to this indirect approach as opposed to a direct suggestions such as, "Today in trance you will no doubt *learn* that you can *remember* many experiences from earlier in life."

Ask the client, "Is it okay if today we induce trance by way of memories you have from earlier in life?" Clients who object to this will let you know reflexively and nonverbally before they answer verbally. For such cases, you should have ready another less threatening induction, perhaps another conversational induction in this chapter. Most clients will not understand what is meant by "inducing trance by way of memories. . . ." We simply tell them, "You will find it interesting, and all you have to do right now is settle into that chair and either close your eyes or just gaze off into the distance, focusing attention on anything you like . . . and just notice your breathing . . . how two deep, refreshing breaths can begin to relax your mind, and your body . . . ."

Induction

(Client's name), people have many, many *things in their experience*, thoughts, memories . . . things they have seen or done throughout their life . . . *words* spoken by us and by others . . . *and* as your mind drifts now . . . you can know that there is nothing that you need to do, or think about, and you can let the words *drift in* and *drift out*, barely paying attention to them at all . . . that's the way . . .

truisms

linking word

apposition of opposites

One person said one time that she thought she could *remember* the day they brought her home from the hospital. Certainly that seems very, very young to be able to *remember* something, anything at all . . . but like I told her then, it really doesn't matter if you *remember* the whole thing or merely a small part of some experience, because the important thing is to just let yourself become more and more more *absorbed* in the experience, letting it happen all by itself. . . .

metaphor

seed (activated)

suggestion

You may have in your mind very vivid and precise memories of certain happy occasions, perhaps when you were very *young*, or maybe as a *teenager*, or *some place in between, any age at all* . . . or even uneventful occasions, and maybe ones that were in no way either happy or uneventful, and any unpleasant or

suggestion covering all possibilities

suggestion

distracting ones can be *conveniently relegated to the background*, not unlike a noise in the hallway . . . that's the way . . . It can be very *interesting* to experience, just *observe inwardly*, what comes up . . . *and* you may find it especially *curious to see* what occurs . . . in there . . . how one thing invariably *leads to another*, all by itself. . . .

implication
pacing
linking word

leading

Birthday parties . . . holiday occasions . . . things you did with others, many, many things . . . things that people did together . . . and places you went . . . and it can be so very pleasant and comfortable to just let your mind *drift and dream*, or *dream and drift* . . . more and more deeply immersed in *one specific memory* . . . or maybe a recollection of *many things blended together* . . . or just a *small piece or fragment* of one thing, like a color or a smell, or just a *nonspecific feeling or overall impression*, or *something else* that perhaps comes and goes, or remains there. . . .

bind of comparable alternatives

suggestion covering all possibilities

One time *a man* thought about his elementary school—I think he referred to it as grammar school—the desks in a straight row, the letters of the alphabet up above the blackboard, or chalkboard . . . I forget which he said . . . and still *another person*, one time she could remember tables and chairs and many other things in the classroom. . . .

metaphor

metaphor

Both of *those people* could still hear, in their heads, "The Alphabet Song," but only one of them could recall hearing classmates singing that song about the wheels on the bus going 'round and 'round . . . . *One person* went to a camp

metaphor

metaphor

in the summer . . . and another attended some kind of religious instruction . . . and both said they could still see the faces of the other kids. . . .

All kinds of experiences . . . I remember *one person* talking about being ten or twelve years old, during the hot days of summer, and passing the time absorbed in her collection of dolls . . . and for another person it was baseball cards . . . things they did during those years. *One woman*, when she was young, growing up in Nebraska—it was a *long, hot*, dry summer—and one afternoon a *short, cold* rain shower happened and she could very vividly recall, even *feel right then*, getting out of the *cold* rain and pressing her back against the *warm* bricks of the building . . . just *absorbed* in the experience. And later she became similarly *immersed* in the Pittsburgh Steelers.

A man named Bru—he walked *fast* with a cane—but he wasn't *slow* in his mind, and he became totally lost *up* there in his mind and *down* there in his body when he played those long, slow songs on the piano on Martha's Vineyard.

As *a young boy*, Toivo swam in the cold, cold waters of Lake Superior and Lake Michigan, and then . . . through the eyes of a child . . . he gazed at the splash of spectacular colors in his father's flower garden. *Lost deeply in thought*, he answered, "Thank you very much," though no one had uttered a word.

As a boy, *David* remembered sleeping on his arm, while the other arm

metaphor

metaphor

apposition of opposites

suggestion

apposition of opposites

suggestions

metaphor
apposition of opposites

metaphor

suggestion

metaphor

was draped over his cat, Binkie, and when he woke up *that* arm was still asleep . . . not unlike what *Kenneth* said about sitting on the tile floor in Walker School, sitting there a long time with your legs crossed and one, or both, of *those* legs, falls deeply asleep. . . .

dissociation
metaphor

Remembering the first time you tasted . . . something . . . sweet . . . or salty. . . . *One person*, Janelle, she could remember way up there in the Upper Penninsula of Michigan, where she came to appreciate Chapstick before lipstick, and it seemed like only yesterday, at the county fair, the experience of eating peanut brittle when she had only a few teeth . . . and now when she has many teeth she can still feel . . . and taste . . . that . . . way back then. . . .

metaphor

Two other people, it happened long, long ago and my memory of it is very dim and hazy, and I think his name was *Clark* and hers was *Tiffany*, and he was telling her late one night about growing up and how he could remember moving from Connecticut to Vermont to New Hampshire, and then *moving again to some other state*, and Clark always *dreamed*, just *dreamed* about growing up and flying on Air Force One, and Tiffany had fantasies about Athens in Greece. . . .

metaphor

suggestion

hypnotic language

Learning to read and write may be blended in with other experiences . . . way back then . . . talking, doing, experiencing when you were young . . . animals or characters in certain picture books. . . . *A woman* once—I think it was Pam over on Glenn Street—said

metaphor

she could remember a big person reading to her ... slowly and deliberately ...
and also remember when she, herself,
began to read . . . and even later when
reading came much more easily . . . all
the way up to the present time . . . when
the word *curmudgeon* still evokes
memories of old Dan. . . . Pam said it can
be very pleasant to become all involved
in talking about nothing because you
forget the specifics but you definitely
remember the nice feeling. . . .   *suggestion*

Deepening

(Client's name), I can only imagine, or otherwise wonder about the
different things you experienced here today. Perhaps there were one
or two or more things that are especially memorable, anything at
all . . . I would like you now to imagine, just imagine, one of those
things that you thought about today, and when that's there, let me
know by nodding your head . . . good . . . and I'd like you now to let
your experience deepen by becoming more and more absorbed in
that *one thing*, taking as much time as you need, and when you feel
your experience has sufficiently deepened, let me know by nodding
your head one more time.

REALERTING

Following therapy, the client may be alerted in the following way: "In
a moment I'm going to ask you to return to your alert state. Before
we do so, I want to recognize the good job that you did here today by
going into trance by just contemplating some things from earlier in
your life. In a few moments I will ask you to share any part of that
experience you would like, recognizing that it is natural to forget
some things. You may now open your eyes and resume your alert
state."

DEBRIEFING

Clients make our job easier by constantly providing us with "gold
nuggets." Debriefing may yield strengths or talents long forgotten, or

a new way to view an old problem. At the very least, this induction provides the therapist with imaginal resources generated during the deepening. Let's say the client reports that her *one thing* was "a sunset on the beach that summer," and that it is a potent and very relaxing image. In future sessions you may take a major shortcut, simply inducing trance by way of absorption in the image.

NOTES FOR PRACTICE

As you develop your own inductions, an early learning set can be easily adapted to particular clients or a specific region. You should include a wide range of common experiences and an array of suggestions, metaphors, and hypnotic phenomena. You may be tempted to provide *specificity* in your script. However, you should allow the client to fill in as many details as possible. For example, instead of saying, "In autumn, you can picture in your mind the burnt red and brilliant yellow leaves that stand out against the powder-blue sky," we prefer you say, "You can imagine . . . in autumn . . . the color of the leaves . . . and the sky. . . ." Too much specificity *restricts* the client's experience. He will likely have difficulty imagining it, and such incongruence lightens trance. On the other hand, clients often find that a general and permissive suggestion stimulates their imagination and can be easily self-referenced. Ample pauses aid clients in retrieving pleasant experiences.

Sometimes a pleasant memory may also be sad. One of my (SB) clients retrieved a pleasant scene and then, reminded of her deceased husband, spontaneously cried. Abreaction may occur at any time during trancework, especially when dealing with memories.

Clients may retrieve a memory and unquestioningly trust its veracity. Accordingly, therapists should discuss how memories may not be valid and how any "memory" may be distortion or fantasy. Clients may also need to be reminded of the goal of hypnotherapy. If the goal has nothing to do with a historical issue such as abuse, pursuing the topic may be needlessly reinforcing an unproductive direction in therapy. Therapists should also be judicious in logging "recovered memories" in the client's record. Practitioners should be familiar with the guidelines of The American Society of Clinical Hypnosis (1995). The risks of inappropriately influencing client memories are minimized when dealt with appropriately.

Other problems with trancework may arise. Some clients with

PTSD, accustomed to chronic muscular and autonomic hyper-arousal, will experience intrusive thoughts or abreaction with hypnosis, or even during conventional progressive muscle relaxation. Evidently, diminished arousal and drops in tension levels send messages that the brain cannot interpret or integrate, resulting in upsetting feelings (Horevitz, 1986). Some personality-disordered or traumatized clients may experience fearful imagery in trance, not because of evoked memories, but because of their need for protection against intrusion. In other words, hypnosis—and the therapist—represent a relationship threat. For some other clients, the hypnotic experience represents an object loss. As they are absorbed in their own inner experience they become frightened because they lose connection with the therapist and the perceived real world. In these situations Horevitz (1986) recommends substituting concrete methods with a low focus on mental activity—progressive muscle relaxation, autogenic relaxation, or biofeedback—or very slow, stepwise use of hypnosis. Clearly, with some clients, it is wise not to use hypnosis at all.

INTERSPERSAL

Inductions in this book thus far have been rather straightforward, designed for clients who show little or no resistance. With the interspersal induction we begin to delve into more elaborate inductions, designed to meet the challenge of chronic and resistant clients. For tough clinical presentations, we often need to try something other than conversational inductions. Two potent and vigorous devices in the "something different" arsenal are embedded meaning and interspersal. Embedded meaning will be treated extensively in the next chapter. We conclude this chapter with an example of interspersal, a highly versatile technique easily adapted to other inductions.

We devised this induction while working with a man we will refer to as Tim. Tim's childhood was uneventful, but as an 18-year-old soldier in Vietnam he went berserk and killed several innocent civilians. Subsequently, the faces of the dead plagued him in regular nightmares. Tim looked much older than his 50 years and his general presentation was one of guilt and shame. At the same time, his speech was filled with words like *duty*, *loyalty*, *honor*, and *respect* for the U.S. and its flag.

The presenting problem, however, was pain from arthritis in his back and various joints. Tim was on a multitude of medications for pain, depression, hypertension, and pulmonary and cardiac problems. A separate interview with his wife revealed that the client was overly preoccupied with his pills. He diligently followed the doctor's orders and had current medications lined up on the kitchen counter. He also insisted on keeping all old medications, including his wife's and children's, and he had hundreds of bottles of pills in the kitchen cupboards. Furthermore, he kept his deceased mother's pills in boxes in the garage. "He has a thousand pill bottles if he has one," remarked his wife.

Tim had eschewed mental health treatment until now, but he was interested in hypnosis for pain management. He declined to say any more about his military service. He did agree that his current strategy was not working, and understood that he needed to do something different. Since he did not respond to general conversational inductions, we devised this interspersal induction around a topic dear to him: pills. In an attempt to join with his rather rigid views, we preceded the interspersal suggestion, "You can do it, Tim," with one of his stated values. Note that we say, "do it different" in the interspersal suggestion because this was how he said it. The concept of "doing things different" is seeded in pre-trance discussion by talking about all the different routes to the hospital and the various parking lots available there. We use interspersal again in the deepening, which is "The Maple Tree."

Induction

One day I saw a woman named Melody, who had a rather interesting problem. "I have to take my pills *differently*," was the way she described her problem. She was taking a particular medication—I forget which one—and for several weeks Melody had taken the pills in this way: one of them three times a day with food. She religiously took one pill with milk and crackers at 8 o'clock, 12 o'clock, and 4 o'clock. Now I never did figure out why it was so important for her to take her pills differently, but that's neither here nor there, as my job is to help people with whatever problem they come in with.

(Doing the *honorable* thing is important, and *you can do it different*, Tim, and you *can* relax both your mind and your body.)

As you may know, many people who make their way to us have already tried many things, and sometimes this therapy business is a last resort. Clients may have attempted every conceivable solution, but they still have not gotten *from here to there*. In Melody's case, she had tried taking half a pill at 8 o'clock, another half at 10 o'clock, and another half at 12 o'clock, 2 o'clock, 4 o'clock, 6 o'clock, and 8 o'clock. She had even tried taking a half at 9 o'clock, 11 o'clock, 1 o'clock, 3 o'clock, 5 o'clock, and 7 o'clock, and she also tried taking half a pill on the half-hour six times a day, and even one-quarter of a pill 12 times a day on both the hour and the half-hour. She even contemplated an eighth of a pill every hour during the day and night, but Melody protested having to get up at night and she added, "Milk and crackers every hour—even in St. Cloud, Minnesota they wouldn't do *that*," and already she was beginning to have concerns about the pill's therapeutic effect.

(*Respect* is important to a man, Tim, and *you can do it different*, and you *can* relax both your mind and your body.)

Eventually Melody and I began to discuss *other ways of getting from here to there*. She came up with many, many new ideas, and I was quite surprised by her resourcefulness. She said that in cutting the pills she could use a different knife and different cutting surface. She had 15 other knives at home and two alternate cutting boards, but then she realized that a variety of other flat surfaces in her apartment would work just fine. The pharmaceutical company had conveniently imprinted its name and the number 23 on the pill. Melody could cut one pill on the "e" and another on the 2, and then a host of other cutting possiblities came to to mind.

(Everyone recognizes the need to *do your duty*, and *you can do it different*, Tim, and you *can* relax both your mind and your body.)

She could also cut those pills during different times of the day, or she could have her mother cut every other pill. She could take one dose in the bathroom and one in the living room and another while driving to work. Instead of milk and crackers she could take juice, and she could have friends present while she took her dose, or maybe play one of her father's old vinyl records. "I could even think different thoughts each time," Melody said, and at that point it was clear to her, and to me, that there was an *infinite number of possibilities of getting from here to there.*

Deepening

Tim, you may let your experience deepen as I tell you another little story now, a story called "The Maple Tree." We can think of trees in our experience, maybe a tree standing alone, perhaps a tree living among other trees, maybe in a vast forest, I don't know, after all, trees are just trees and I've always wondered why people make so much of trees, likening the mighty oak to who-knows-what, I can only imagine . . . (*you can go deep*). At any rate, not so long ago, it was a blustery autumn in a forest, in a grove of ordinary maple trees, where the crows cawed up above and lower down squirrels jumped from tree to tree.

Seeds were blowing down from the maple trees, (*you can go deep*) and like most seeds, the vast majority of them didn't sprout or take root but got eaten or just decomposed on the floor of the forest. But one seed landed on an old log (*you can go deep*) and just stayed there, and eventually it became covered by the snows of winter, and there it lay, unnoticed by deer and rabbits.

In the spring, the seed was still there. It swelled with moisture and sprouted and a tiny root creeped down into the damp, rich, rotting wood of the old log. And slowly it grew, a seedling, with scrawny branches and little green leaves that stretched toward the sun. And it continued to grow, and the years passed, (*you can go deep*) and the rich and fertile soil allowed it to survive drought, and somehow the animals never ate it, and two times during a forest fire rain blew in and saved it at the last minute.

In the fall this mature tree's green leaves turned a yellow orange and then a burning red. In the winter, the maple tree slept, just like all the other trees, and just like insects in the logs and chipmunks underground, dormant, resting for the winter. Birds sat up high in the tall branches (*you can go deep*) and winter continued on. One day, the unbearable weight of the snow caused a huge branch to break off. The sharp sound cracked through the forest. But then spring comes and green leaves come out again and sap flows through the tree. Bees and insects and birds live in and around the tree, and animals run down below.

One summer day, a bolt of lightning crashes into the tree and splits it up near the top, but the seasons continue on, and the tree continued to put out seeds of its own, and the roots thrust *deep in the soil*, roots intermingled with other roots, *deep* below the ground.

REALERTING

Tim was realerted quickly to facilitate amnesia: "You may wake up right now, Tim!" Sometimes people with pain are distracted by their discomfort and have trouble remaining still during trancework. However, Tim appeared deep in trance as he showed facial mask, very little swallowing, and minimal movement in his chair.

DEBRIEFING

When asked how he felt, he said, "I didn't feel anything, but I don't remember anything either." His response was positive for time distortion and numbness in his hands and feet in addition to amnesia. "I don't have much pain right now," he added. He was reinforced for his positive response, and he indicated eagerness to continue next time.

NOTES FOR PRACTICE

After Tim's good inital response, he cancelled two appointments in a row and was eventually lost to follow-up. When this happens we always wonder: Did I (GG) not pay enough attention to control issues? What did I miss? Did he get scared off by my interest in his possible PTSD? Certainly the future plan was to refer him to the PTSD specialists at the clinic. Viewing a videotape of the session or discussing the case in supervision or in a team meeting can be helpful. However, like all therapists, we have cases where we can only wonder what went wrong.

The bright side of Tim's case was that we learned the importance of utilizing a client's preoccupation as a device for inducing trance. We have since induced trance by utilizing similar problematic pursuits such as cleaning house, making a good impression, or "coming out on top." Notice that the above induction employed only one suggestion for trance, which was repeated following each interspersal. The induction route, or means for absorbing Tim's attention, was pills. In developing your own inductions for clients who do not respond to conversational inductions, we suggest you pay attention to salient aspects of their presentation. A client's strong interest in something nonproblematic may lack sufficient potency to absorb attention. Instead, we suggest you look for an aspect of the problem that is repetitive and strongly maintains the status quo.

We regularly employ both "Pills" and "The Maple Tree" without interspersal for ego-strengthening in therapy. In some ways, interspersal is a more versatile device than embedded meaning, which often requires more knowledge and preparation ahead of time. One advantage of embedded meaning (as well as truisms, bind of comparable alternatives, and other hypnotic techniques) is that you can employ it in standard talk therapy, while interspersal requires trance. Interspersal suggestions can be inserted at any point in an induction or story. A good rule with interspersal is to *keep it simple*. Rather than mixing suggestions, it is best to stick with one (*you can go deep*), whose potency is derived from repetition and vocal change. You don't want to overdo it. Like utilization and other concepts, less may be more. Some practitioners employ interspersal *not* as a non-sequitur within a story, but rather as a natural part of the story, subtly highlighted by a pause and vocal change. For further reading on interspersal, see Erickson's complete works (Rossi, 1980).

We let clients know ahead of time that we will be telling them a story interspersed with suggestions. That knowledge does not diminish the effectiveness of a very potent technique. In fact, it may become *more* effective because you are respecting the client's right to know—even in general terms—what to expect in the session.

3

Embedded-Meaning
Inductions

THE ROAD

This induction arose from a discussion with one of our interns whose client wanted to experience trance but had some reservations about doing so. The client had a negative experience several years earlier when her therapist had tried—unsuccessfully—to induce trance with an eye roll induction. She had found this intrusive and overly directive. Not only did she fail to go into trance, she also failed to return for a second session.

The client related that she had experienced naturalistic trance through "losing myself" while driving her car. Accordingly, she responded well to the following induction, as have innumerable other clients who appreciate an induction that capitalizes on an ordinary, everyday experience. Such experiences lend themselves to embedded meaning.

We soon learned that, in addition to readily inducing trance, such embedded meaning inductions have the useful byproduct of ego-strengthening. Hartland (1971) believed that many clients will not give up their symptoms until they are strong enough to do so. He likened many mental health clients to debilitated medical patients who must undergo surgery. In order to do well after surgery, it may be necessary to strengthen them through proper rest and nutrition beforehand. "Building clients up" early in therapy may properly prepare them for subsequent hypnotherapeutic interventions.

Authoritarian approaches to ego-strengthening involve repeated, direct suggestions in trance such as "You *can* be strong" or "You *can* overcome this problem." Such an approach may be useful with clients who require considerable directiveness, but most clients evidence greater benefit from a more respectful, indirect practice. This type of approach presumes that clients have the inherent ability to solve their own problems and are seeking a gentle nudge from the therapist, who has contracted to use metaphor and story to access their unconscious mind and get in "underneath the radar." Inevitably, clients self-reference the metaphor, or meta-message.

Many who have done this induction practice with seeding during pre-induction discussion. They may, for example, casually mention that they *noticed* something in the morning newspaper, on the evening news, or on the freeway yesterday. Accordingly, the idea of *notice* is later activated when it appears in the induction. *Notice* and *appreciate*, two key hypnotic talents to be bolstered in all clients, are inextricably linked in this and other inductions.

You will notice the word *fluff* appearing in the right-hand column. Why fluff? Because any induction or therapeutic story needs boring or meaningless material to distract the listener's conscious mind. Often inductions or stories become too purposeful or didactic. Follow the law of parsimony instead: Less is more. Couching suggestions in fluff may make them more effective.

Induction

Everyone knows what it's like to be driving down the road, feeling the warm sun shining through the window on a cold day, or on a hot day, *experiencing a refreshing breeze* when you roll down that window. The *warm sun*, a *cool*	*truism*
	naturalistic trance experiences

breeze, or the *rhythm of traffic*—all that is something that people can become *absorbed in one way*, or *immersed in some other way*, paying attention to *just one thing*, or to *nothing in particular*, or perhaps they just allow their *minds to drift off. . . .*

bind of comparable alternatives

You *speed up* and *slow down*, and sometimes you can drift to a stop at *that* light, almost without thinking, and other times you will purposely apply the brake hard to make a sharp turn off the road. It is interesting how you will *slow down* to 15 miles per hour in a school zone, and a few moments later you might be going at high speed down the interstate. People from out of town might creep along aggravatingly slow, and we know how some teenagers drive. One man one time said he *needed new brakes* once a year, and another said his brake pedal *still looked new* after five years of city driving. Whether you're talking about a *heavy foot* or a *light foot*, both of *those* feet seem to operate *all by themselves, independently*, or with *their own autonomy*, or almost like they're *detached* from the drivers' legs, strange as that might seem. Of course, even thinking about all that may be part of *slowing down*.

apposition of opposites

dissociative language

suggestion

fluff

apposition of opposites

dissociative language

suggestion

It's interesting to *notice* how many times a person gets in that car, sits behind the wheel, starts the engine, and begins to drive down the road, just like other people going from here to there. Your hands—and your feet—do the job effortlessly, *without even thinking*, and your mind can sometimes get

seeding (activated)

involuntariness

lost in the music, the scenery, or all the other things that you *notice* and come to *appreciate* going down the road.

seeding

Time can seem to *speed up*, or *slow down*, or maybe while you're behind the wheel you're simply *unaware of the passage of time.* On a car's clock, or on your watch, a *minute* can seem like an *hour*, or an *hour* can seem like a *minute*, but it *really doesn't matter* because all you have to do is sit behind the wheel. I knew *a woman* one time whose left foot would always fall asleep, and another who learned to pay particular attention to how many deep breaths she could get in while waiting for that long traffic light to change.

bind of comparable alternatives

time distortion

not knowing/not doing

metaphor

Someone one time said that once she came to *notice* all these things, a short time later she came to *appreciate* everything whether it was time being *fast* or *slow*, or whether it was a *heaviness* or *lightness* or some other sensation in her extremities, or somewhere else. *Noticing and appreciating* just went together, not unlike on the road where you see a *tractor* and a *trailer*, or *one* lane running alongside *another* lane, or *two* tires on one side balanced by *two* tires on the other side, or a turn signal for *both directions*, or a person driving and *one* in the passenger seat, and maybe *two* in the front and *two* in the back.

seeding (activated)

apposition of opposites

seeding (activated)

metaphor

A woman one time—I think it was Judy from Neptune City, New Jersey— said that she *learned a lot* while waiting for that light to change, just by looking in the rearview mirror. She found it

metaphor

very *curious* that the woman in the | *hypnotic language*
rearview mirror behind her was mouth-
ing the words to the song that she also
had on the radio, and so did the man in
the side mirror off to the left. Actually,
for days later, she continued to *wonder*. | *hypnotic language*
Another time on a very cold morning,
she *noticed* that the exhaust from her | *seeding* (activated)
car danced and lingered in the air
exactly the same as the exhaust from
the other cars. She thought, "How
interesting! Am I the only one who | *hypnotic language*
notices these things?"

A very *careful and conscientious driver*, she always stayed between the lines, which can't be said for every *fluff* driver on the road. *Looking at the car ahead*—or the car behind—she learned to anticipate whether those vehicles were going to turn right or turn left, long before the driver signalled intent. She wondered what it was that allowed her to predict this with near one-hundred percent accuracy. *Was it because* *fluff* the drivers slowed down imperceptibly, or because they leaned ever so slightly in that direction before they made their turn? She still doesn't know for sure, but she continues to *notice* and study many *seeding* (activated) interesting phenomena of the road.

One day, waiting for a light to change, her *mind wandered* and she *wondered* *hypnotic language* about her friend back in Iowa who bragged about her ability to start her car on a cold day, and she had responded to her friend that she knew how to *keep her car cool* in the Arizona sun. When she was *driving back there* in *fluff* Iowa one summer, looking for her friend's house, her friend had told her to "turn left where the sign for the church used to be," and *she was proud* that she had found her friend's house anyway. She thought about everything involved in *negotiating all kinds of traffic*, going safely *from here to there, finding her way* on unfamiliar roads, and, of course, *finding your way* while driving at night can be *something to feel very proud about*.

ego-strengthening

That same woman, one time, was describing her 90-year-old grandfather who had kept the *same Chevrolet* for 39 years and it had only 50,000 miles on it and *not a speck of rust*. Her grandfather talked about having had a string of bad luck for a long time and he sat her down once when she was young and said that *on any road* a person will run into *potholes* and have occasional *flat tires and fender benders, maybe even major accidents*, but he told her the road is always there and that *you will get back on* it, and that the good stuff way down the road might come soon or might take a while, but that the important thing was that you *continue to get back on the road*. And the woman said she *appreciated* that story and that eventually she came to really *notice* all the other people on the road, too.

fluff

metaphor

ego-strengthening

seeding (activated)

Getting out on the open road, a person sees a lot, and everyone needs time to look around outside as well as *inside*. Being aware of blind spots might take some doing, no matter what kind of mirrors these vehicles have. Good clear views of the sides and rear are possible,

suggestion

especially on a clear day. But if you're
going down the freeway, in the *middle
lane*, watching the *car ahead* is most
important, but then there's the *car
behind*, and traffic on each side. Now
that's four things to try and pay attention to, and while all that's going on, a
person is always thinking, or listening
to the radio, or *watching for something
alongside the road*, or traffic coming
from the other direction. With so many
things to look at out there, it can be
very comfortable and satisfying to
notice what comes from inside. Now
parallel parking, some people have difficulty doing that, but they have to just
do it because nobody's invented a mirror yet to show you the right front. Just
finding any parking place is tough
sometimes, and they're always telling
you, "DON'T PARK HERE!" which is
just another thing that you have to
notice and get accustomed to, but you
can probably remember how utterly
frustrating it can be finding a place,
but eventually you always find one
somewhere.

Driving a long distance is something
everybody knows about, and there's
always some anticipation or uncertainty when starting out on a long trip.
I remember once *a man* telling me
about getting ready for a long trip.
Other people, before a long trip, might
be sure to check the tires, and check to
see if they have *road flares and things
like that*, but this man, he wasn't always
on top of things like he should be, and
he just set out down the road with little

fluff

suggestion

seeding (activated)

metaphor

fluff

thought or preparation, going from Phoenix to San Diego, which is hardly a day-long journey. The words still rang in his head. Were they the words of his father or somebody else? *"Your spare*   *fluff* *tire is the most important tire on your car,"* were the exact words.

And sure enough, when a tire went flat out on the road when he least expected it, he discovered that the spare was also flat. So, it took more time and trouble to get where he was going, but he got there just the same. Now going between Phoenix and San Diego is a lot of straight, *monotonous* freeway, through barren desert and a few sand dunes, not much at all to see or do, an occasional small town, and driving along *your mind just drifts*, and it's very easy to become absorbed in the lines of the road, almost like getting *lulled to sleep*, where you become *obliv-*   *suggestions* *ious to time*, and although you're driving down the road, it's like you're float-ing along on autopilot, with your mind—or your body—*detached, or not*   *dissociation* *connected* to anything in particular.

Now this man, as he went down the road he was lost in *wondering* about   *hypnotic language* this and that and *imagining* many things. He didn't notice that he was climbing a steady grade into the moun-tains. Signs along the road warned drivers to turn off their *air conditioners* to avoid overheating, and eventually overheat is what he did, and he had to   *fluff* pull off the road. With some patience and the passage of time the *radiator cooled* down, and water was near, which he was very thankful for, and he continued on down the road, paying much better attention now.

As he was telling me this I *lost track of time* and lost track of whether there was any point to what he was telling me, but after listening closely for a while I figured that it *didn't really matter* anyway, and *I would pick up* any meaning or importance one way or the other, as *I often did two or more things* at a time, and was *proud* that in the end everything got done and I *felt really good* about myself.

time distortion

not knowing/not doing

ego-strengthening

Now this man, after cooling down his car, he continued on, a bit wiser now about the signs along the road. I can't remember if he said his *hand* became *numb* on the wheel, or if his *foot fell asleep*, or if he simply *felt immobile* there behind the wheel, just driving along, but he definitely remembered it as a very pleasant and curious experience.

suggestions

As he got closer to San Diego he began to *dream* about the beach and wind blowing through the palms. Perhaps he was going faster than he should have but he still was able to read a sign as he went by, and the sign warned of high winds the next ten miles, so he instinctively slowed down, and just then his car was buffeted by a gust of wind. He squeezed the steering wheel and *held the car steady* in his lane, and other strong gusts continued to blow his car, and never once did he let it stray into the other lane, and he *felt quite good about how he had handled that strong, strong wind.*

hypnotic language

suggestion

ego-strengthening

(If clients have not already closed their eyes, you may say something like, "You may now let your eyes gently close," and if they keep their eyes open, simply pace the behavior with "You may find it comfortable to just let yourself become absorbed in some spot out there.")

Deepening

I'm going to be quiet for a few moments and during that time I would like you to imagine, just imagine yourself sinking deeper and deeper into a very pleasant state of relaxation, and when you are sufficiently deep, you will know and I will know because you will find yourself taking two nice, deep breaths.

REALERTING

Following the therapy portion, the client may be realerted in the following manner, which emphasizes time distortion (a hypnotic phenomenon that is a strong ratifier of trance): "I'm going to count now from one up to five, and when I get up to five you may open your eyes. When you open your eyes, without looking at your watch, please take a guess at how much time has passed here today. One, two . . ."

DEBRIEFING

Debriefing may include specific questions directed at dissociation, ideosensory feeling, or other hypnotic experience suggested in the induction. Questions can also be more general, such as "How did you feel?" or "What are you thinking about now?" It is important to allow clients time to verbally process their experience.

NOTES FOR PRACTICE

We often use some aspect of *driving* or *the road* as an induction or therapeutic story. Just as movement, volition, and progress are central to individual development and psychotherapy, these concepts or processes are common to everybody's experience and can be utilized by the therapist. Many aspects of driving, for instance, "being in the driver's seat," symbolize control and mastery for the client. People who have lost their ability to walk or drive may even self-reference a story such as this more strongly than able persons. As this induction is fairly long, you may choose to use only a portion of it, especially if the client has previously experienced trance. Additionally, you may have noticed something in your own driving experience.

A broad metaphor like the road can incorporate a host of therapeutic targets: internal exploration, slowing down, seeding—and activating—behaviors like *noticing*, and enhancing mastery or self-control. Inspiring hope and framing therapy as a process wherein the client is in charge are other helpful outcomes. We use this induction early in therapy to assess capacity for absorption in a story. Sometimes we will ask clients to pay attention to the story and tell us afterward what they *noticed* about their breathing or what learning resulted as part of the process. Of course, "man" or "he" may be substituted for "woman" or "she." However, it is not necessary to precisely "fit" the people in the story to your client. A young female client whom you are treating in Miami may have no difficulty self-referencing a story character who is an older adult male in Seattle. In reading the induction, you may wish to insert pauses, emphasize italicized words, or accent other words, depending on the situation.

Many of the inductions and deepenings in this book lend themselves to mixing and matching—as well as adding or deleting material—depending on client needs and therapist interests. For clients who readily evidence depth in trance, formal deepening may not be necessary. We see deepening as a useful entity for those who are learning hypnosis, as it is a convenient bridge between induction and therapy. For experienced practitioners, deepening is a versatile device in which stories and a variety of other means are employed to both deepen trance and offer suggestions. Used in this way, deepening accelerates hypnotherapy. Critics of deepening believe that therapists should foster creative associations *laterally* rather than deeply and that desired depth in trance may be illusive to both therapists and clients when formal deepening is suggested (Brent Geary, personal communication, 1999). We suggest you experiment with both ways to see what works for you and your clients. Many clients, when queried after trancework, are unable to distinguish deepening as a separate part of the process.

DISSOCIATION

Dissociation is a cardinal feature of hypnosis and is usually included in the definition of hypnosis. Kingsbury (1988) referred to hypnosis as an "isomorphic intervention" for treating posttraumatic stress disorder (PTSD), because dissociation is part of both the artificial state of hypnosis and the pathological state of PTSD. It then follows that an induction that facilitates dissociation—even in clients who sometimes experience dissociation as part of a psychiatric disorder—may be very useful in the repertoire of the hypnotherapist. Association, with complaints, such as chronic pain or anxiety, can be quite problematic. One strategy in treating both of these problems is to assist clients in *dis*sociating from them.

Like the other inductions in this book, this one draws on ordinary experiences. Dissociation occurs with a wide variety of everyday experience. We have found that people are suggestible to metaphors using common experiences, involving people to whom they can relate. This metaphorical approach is especially helpful with clinical populations such as older adults (Gafner, 1997), patients with psychotic disorders (Gafner & Young, 1998), and other clients not traditionally treated with hypnotherapy. It has a host of advantages, in that it allows the therapist to bypass reflexive objections of clients, tests clients' responses to ideas without calling attention to them, and builds a strong, unseen foundation before becoming overt. Using metaphor to dissociate also encourages clients' internal search for stored or imagined resources and creates new associative pathways. Accordingly, clients may experience a greater sense of creativity in, and responsibility for, the therapy process (Combs & Freedman, 1990).

Dissociation is embedded in this induction in a variety of ways. In keeping with the spirit of dissociation, we have severed the explanation of terms in the right-hand column. You will be able to recognize words like *separate*, *independence*, and *autonomy* as suggestions for dissociation and the associated experiences of amnesia, numbness, and involuntariness. We like to experiment vocally with these highlighted words. Perhaps one time we will emphasize them with a slightly deeper or slower intonation. Other times we won't accent them at all.

As clients make themselves comfortable, we explain that the story they are about to listen to might not make sense, which is okay, because it has been designed to bypass their conscious mind, or "to get in underneath your radar." We tell them that they can either listen to it or just let the words drift in and drift out.

Induction

We have all had many experiences, some that were memorable, some not so, some that were pleasant and good, and others that we *may not recall*. Just like dreams, everyone has had them, and many we *forget by the time we wake up*, and other times we may remember only a small part of that dream.

One time I slept on my right arm most of the night, and that arm was *still asleep* long after I woke up. That was similar to when my left leg *fell asleep* when I was sitting down, and after I got up to walk the leg still had a strong tingling sensation, or maybe it was just *a numbness*, I *forget*.

I remember back in grade school a teacher said, "*It's your ears* I'm speaking to," which seemed rather curious at the time, how your ears could be *separated* from the rest of you. When the teacher was speaking I would often just drift off, maybe listening to a word here or a word there, sometimes paying attention to this or that, and when she would look at me—or maybe it was the person next to me—I would snap out of it for a moment or two, and then I would resume daydreaming. One time in class I remember that I was sitting on a chair behind the table, legs crossed, and sometimes one leg would *fall asleep* as I drifted off, and one time both legs *fell asleep*, which can be very different from the kind of *detachment* a person feels when absorbed in a movie, or some other interesting experience when you *lose* track of time. One time I had my hand raised, way up in the air, because I wanted to answer the teacher's question, and *that hand* just stayed up there, in the air, *on its own*, for the longest time. . . .

That same teacher would often tell us stories. I don't know what she intended by all those stories, and I must admit, lots of times I didn't catch her drift, and from *what I can remember*, she would usually start out those stories by saying, "Today I'll be speaking to *your third ear*." Yes, *third ear* is what she actually said, which I wonder about to this day, and I can still hear her voice.

One day the teacher was telling us about someone she knew—I think she called her Dorothy. Years ago it had happened, and even today I can *recall only a portion* of this story. Dorothy was a young girl then and it happened in another state, *away from the city*, and there was forest all around, and Dorothy had *lost* her purse along a country road. Somehow it *fell out* of the car, and the car moved on, and *time and distance separated her from that purse*. It was probably a matter of hours—and some minutes—before she went back to look for it, riding a bicycle, and by then it was very late in the afternoon. Up ahead on the road she saw her purse, and by now she was deep in the woods and her legs were so tired from pedaling that they had *hardly any feeling* in them at all. As she eagerly bent down to pick it up, the purse seemed to assume *a life of its own* as it suddenly *jerked away* from her grasp. Some children had yanked it away on a string, simply a prank, but she always wondered what those children were doing way out there. She eventually got her purse back, minus a few dollars, which she didn't mind a bit.

Riding back down that country road, she held her purse tightly, *out there* on the handle bar whose grip on the right side had fallen off, and a spoke *was missing* on the front wheel, although she didn't notice these things until much later. By now it was growing increasingly dark, and her rate of breathing had changed considerably. She couldn't see much behind her, or ahead of her for that matter. If she held her hand *out in front of her* face she could barely see it. She slowed down on that road, feet moving on the pedals *all by themselves*, and it was almost as if *those feet belonged to somebody else*, and as she looked down at her feet she *could not remember* an evening quite as dark as this one. Had it not been a familiar road, it would have been easy to *lose her way*.

Dorothy continued down the road of life. One evening at the state fair she ate cotton candy and salt water taffy, but not at the same time. She remembered *pulling apart* a piece of salt water taffy, long and slow, and the sweetness dissolved in her mouth slowly, but not as quickly as the cotton candy, which she ate faster. She *didn't even realize* she was down to the paper cone and then she noticed all the little sugar crystals in the last gauze of sweetness, way too many little crystals to count even if she would have bothered to do so.

In a high school class Dorothy wrote a report on the *separation* of church and state, and somehow this reminded her of the chain on her bike, not the chain to lock up her bike, but rather the chain that propelled her forward, each vital segment linked to the next, and of course, with any chain, if one section *becomes separated* from the piece in front, or the piece in back, a *disconnection* occurs, which is something a person realizes sooner rather than later.

After college Dorothy worked as an engineer for one of the smaller oil companies, which grew bigger with the passage of time, and eventually its stock *split two for one*, and then the company *broke away* from its parent company and became its own entity, and later it merged with yet another company, but the merger was challenged by the attorneys who argued that a law had *been broken*. They questioned whether the spirit—if not the letter—of some law had been *breached*, but through it all Dorothy kept her job. She appreciated the fact that they let her work very *independently*.

At work, Dorothy had a good deal of *autonomy* and she would sometimes become inattentive or distracted, for example, becoming immersed or absorbed in things like how water *can be separated* into hydrogen and oxygen, or *the separation* of molecules or electrolytes into *constituent parts*, or isolating or extracting something from a compound or mixture, or even more everyday things like *how oil separates from water*, or a fork in the road, or the meaning of a wall—or a fence—that *separates one house from another*. This got her thinking about a whole range of concepts involving space and time, as well as imaginary connections or dotted lines on her company's organizational chart.

But time for Dorothy, as she continued down that road, went on slowly, and sometimes quickly. The longer she went on, she realized that time on a clock did not matter much anyway. Many things *left behind* were now just pleasant memories, or *forgotten about altogether*.

Deepening

(You may suggest eye closure if the client's eyes are still open, or simply pace continued eye fixation.) Now I'd like you to count silently to yourself, down from twenty to one, slowly, taking as much time as you need, and when you have reached one it will be a signal to you that you are in a very comfortable state of trance, and let me know when you're there by nodding your head. You may start to count silently now. . . .

REALERTING

Following the therapy portion, you may realert the client by counting from one to five, asking the client to reawaken "at your own pace," or employing a similar method for gentle realerting.

DEBRIEFING

You may wish to experiment with a double bind question when clients open their eyes. For instance, asking, "Are you still in trance?" may ratify trance as much as other debriefing questions. Whether clients answer yes or no, they must contemplate the extent to which they were in trance.

NOTES FOR PRACTICE

Some clients may experience heightened dissociation as a frightening loss of control. Most of these clients will decline the offer of hypnosis in the first place. Others—including some with severe psychopathology—respond well to this and other inductions. Many of these clients are very good at "spacing out," and sometimes debriefing will yield useful material for next session. For example, during this induction, one client, who had a history of sexual abuse between the ages six and twelve, recalled the pleasant experience of caressing her kitten. "My hand just kept moving, all by itself," she said. She was able to cull this very positive experience from a time in her life that was sad and traumatic. Accordingly, in subsequent sessions she was able to split off the pleasant experience that we used both for deepening ("Imagine yourself now becoming more and more absorbed in caressing your kitten . . . "), as well as a segment of therapy where caressing the kitten on an imagined TV screen gradually enlarged in proportion to a traumatic image on the same screen.

Some clients with personality disorders, severe PTSD, or psychotic disorders may respond more positively if you begin with an induction from Chapter 2 of this book. With all clients, successful therapy results from trust and rapport; clients' positive response builds over time. In clients with severe psychopathology, this vital alliance should be nurtured gradually and slowly. Beginning with a less intricate induction may serve this purpose.

In the Stress Management Program at the Tucson V.A., we begin with the eye fixation induction. More than half of these clients are referred from the Psychotic Disorders Clinic. No hypnosis is done during the first session. When hypnosis begins in the second session, we always bring clients in and out of trance two or three times, thus fostering their sense of control. Following the general and permissive conversational induction used in the first session, they know what to expect, and we can see how they respond. Most who respond favorably to a conversational induction will also respond well to an embedded meaning induction such as the dissociation induction.

TRAVEL

Many people travel by commercial airliner and can relate to the experience as a pedestrian facet of everyday life. Common, ordinary, and even boring experiences may be best suited for hypnotic inductions, as we have found that adults of all ages—and even many adolescents—are more likely to become absorbed in an induction that involves the commonplace, rather than an induction with an enchanted forest, New Age healing crystals, or fantasy figures floating on a cloud above a magic kingdom. An induction with an everyday topic or theme is disarming and innocent and tends to lull people into trance. Of course, enchanted forests may have the same effect on some people, and we apologize if you are disappointed that we included none of those in this book.

Deepening is embedded at the end of this induction, followed by a double deepening in which clients are asked to deepen their experience, lighten it, and then go deep a second time. Embedded meaning and key suggestions are highlighted for vocal emphasis.

Induction

One day I was flying on American Airlines and I don't know if it was a matter of becoming fascinated by or *absorbed in* what was going on during the descent of that airplane. At any rate, I'll never forget that day.

As that airliner began its descent into Dallas-Fort Worth, I thought about being down on the ground, and during those moments time can seem to *speed up* or *slow down*, or maybe you just lose track of time altogether, I don't know. They had just announced that it was time to put on your seat belt and put up the tray table, but I kept my tray table down anyway, even though the person next to me promptly raised his tray table and put away the book he was reading. I continued studying a road map, *out there* on the tray table, examining details of my final destination *down there* on the ground. I thought briefly of putting on my seat belt, but I didn't do that until much later, long after everyone else had done so. It was very interesting to notice just then that my hand had fallen asleep *out there*, off to the side, on the armrest. The numbness had already spread up my arm, but I soon turned my attention to other things.

We were now closer to the ground and as I looked *out there* from *inside*, things down there became clearer the lower we got. I adjusted the map with my one useful hand, as the other one was *so numb*, and then the flight attendant—her voice seemed to *drift in and then drift out*—began to announce connecting gate information: "Abilene, gate 36; Albuquerque, gate 41; Amarillo, gate 37 . . ." and I thought, "I'm going to Sacramento, so I've got lots of time before she gets to the Ss," and at that point I just tuned her out as she continued with Austin and Bakersfield and all the others in alphabetical order.

The passenger in the next seat saw what I was doing and he said, "Don't worry. There's *nothing to know and you don't have to do anything either*," and I still wonder what he meant by that, but at that moment I just drifted off a bit more, into the map in front of me, as the plane continued its descent.

Initially looking at any map it can be difficult to orient yourself among the tangle of colored lines going in every direction. The rivers are blue lines, and the state roads are one thing, and the interstate highways are something else. The broken lines show the county lines, and there appeared to be all solid lines between the states, but on any map it's all too easy to rapidly *drift from one state to another*. A person gets a different point of view, descending in a plane, or studying a map, just being *detached* from it all, kind of like children—and they all do this sooner or later—who bend over and look at the world from between their legs. I would get light-headed if I did that now, and I still remember being in that classroom years before, holding my hand in the air *for the longest time*, but I can't recall if that was my numb hand or the other one.

I turned back to the voice overhead and she had only gotten to the Cs: Carlsbad, gate 35; Colorado Springs, gate 40 . . . and the man next to me—the voice was in a tunnel far away—he said, *"You don't even have to listen,"* and I immediately returned to my map. Turkey Hollow was a strange name, but no more unusual than *Deep* Hollow. Both places you'd probably miss if you blinked or just closed your eyes going by. *In*spiration Point reminded me of breathing, or maybe imagination, I don't know, but *Explore*rs' Post just seemed like something remote. Wilderness *Retreat lacks* something as far as names go, and *In*skeep Corners just sounded like something very remote, perhaps a good place to spend some time. *Slow*poke Ridge probably overlooked a small canyon or ravine down there, and just then the voice overhead announced, "San Jose, gate 29."

I finally put up my tray table and buckled the seat belt with the one hand available to me. Things on the ground were rapidly coming into focus, and the man in the next seat was sitting back, eyes closed. I knew it was time to begin counting silently to myself, down from ten to one. I felt very, very comfortable as the descent continued.

Deepening

(Client's name), in a moment I'm going to count down from ten to one and I'd like you to experience greater depth of trance as each number descends, starting to count now, ten, nine, etc. (After reaching one): Going back up to five . . . *and then* back down once again, letting yourself go deeper and deeper, five, four, three, two, and one.

REALERTING

The client is realerted as described in previous inductions.

DEBRIEFING

During the first few sessions of trancework you should carefully elicit trance ratifiers. Numbness and time distortion are likely convincers in this induction, and people frequently recollect old thoughts and feelings. Travel and geographic markers seem to stimulate this.

NOTES FOR PRACTICE

Sometimes before beginning the induction we forget to ask clients if they feel fearful about flying or airports. If you forget to ask, many clients will reflexively open their eyes and ask you to stop, while more passive clients may show eye flutter. Others may signal their discomfort by shifting anxiously in their chair. If you notice such nonverbals, it may be best to stop immediately and ask for a verbal report of subjective experience. We once had a client who demonstrated such discomfort. When asked what she was feeling, she said, "I'm not sure . . . it's better now." She was told to let her experience deepen during a few moments of silence, and then we continued with the induction, which went quite well from that point on.

We have had several clients who strongly prefer this induction, so we use it with them every time. The double deepening is an eminently effective device, akin to inducing trance and having them come out before going in again. It is often used early in trancework to enhance self-control. The client invariably sinks deeper into trance with the second deepening.

TIME

The concept of time is experienced universally but in myriad ways. It is used as a standard component in hypnotic inductions, and time distortion is a key ratifier of trance. Techniques such as age regression and age progression rely on time. Countless inductions could be developed based on this dominant, pervasive aspect of everyday life.

We have found embedded-meaning inductions, such as the Time induction, very effective with both resistant and non-resistant clients. Non-resistant clients, who will likely go into trance without regard to the induction employed, seem to appreciate opportunities to stimulate their imaginations. Many resistant clients are disarmed by these inductions' casual, innocent non-direction. In other words, they are not presented with anything to consciously resist, and so often incorporate the metaphor, or meta-message, effortlessly.

Age regression is used for deepening, but it is prudent to first ask clients if they are comfortable with such techniques. For example, "In the deepening portion of trancework today I'm going to ask you to drift back in time to some point where you felt pleasantly relaxed. Is that okay?" If the answer is no, clients may be alerting us to a trauma or some other unpleasant experience in their background that they prefer not to revisit. If this is the case, another deepening may be substituted.

Clients are asked to settle in, take two deep refreshing breaths, and either let their eyes gently close or simply fix their gaze on anything in the room.

Induction

Time, as we know it, is something that we often think about, and clock time can be a very *interesting* phenomenon, something that people often *imagine* ... or *wonder* about.	*truism* *hypnotic language*
Now, (client's name), time on a clock, in trance, might seem to *slow down* for some people, and for others it *speeds up*, but for many they simply *don't notice*, or *don't care*, or are *oblivious* to it, perhaps just losing track of time altogether.	*apposition of opposites* *bind of comparable alternatives*
One time a *man* imagined how a *minute* can seem like an *hour*, or an *hour* like a *minute*. Of course, clock time and time in trance are not unlike an *entrance into another state*, and none of this probably matters at all anyway, mere temporal experiences that they are.	*metaphor* *apposition of opposites* *embedded meaning suggestion*
Flying on a long trip, a *person* goes through time zones. On any long trip people *don't have to* do anything at all. They can just sit back and they *don't have to* listen to anything or pay attention to anything, just enjoying the experience. *I* remember once, looking at a map, becoming *absorbed* in those time zones, and *imagining* going from one to another . . . but it may be that actually flying through them *a person* feels more detachment, like when you sit down anywhere for a long time and your *foot*, or your *arm*, can just *fall asleep*, which is different from looking at any one thing for a long time, like a world map, and all those time zones,	*metaphor* *not knowing/not doing* *suggestion* *hypnotic language* *metaphor* *suggestion*

part of you becomes absorbed in the
map and *part of you* just observes or
enjoys the experience.

dissociation

Richard Feynman, the famous physi-
cist, could look at a clock and then
have a *conversation* or *read a book*, or
do something else, for ten or fifteen
minutes or more, and at any point he
could *just stop* and without looking at
his watch he *could tell you* the exact
time, nearly down to the second. Now I
don't know if that has anything or not
to do with dual experience in trance,
where part of the person is in trance
and part of the person just observes the
process, but it *can't not* have to do with
the hidden observer's *in*tuition or
imagi*n*ation, or the mind's special ability to *wonder*, or *wander*, and maybe at
the same time.

metaphor

fluff

double negative
embedded meaning

suggestion

One psychologist here, Bob, said he
told *his brother back in Iowa* that he
couldn't walk and chew gum at the
same time. I don't know about that, but
I *could never concentrate* on two things
at once, so I just quit trying, which is
*in*herently a*kin* to the experience of
one of our psychologists, Deborah *Ing*-
ham-*In*ch, who *entered* through that
door many times, and casually remarked how this entire process may be
a matter of *letting go of control*, or *controlling letting go*, but never both at the
same time, and how all this could be
interpreted as being in the *driver's seat*,
which we all know is very, very comfortable . . . and perhaps incontrovert-
ible *evidence* that letting go is a pleasant experience, which has nothing at
all to do with being in a *convertible*.

fluff

embedded meaning

bind of comparable
alternatives

metaphor

fluff

When a commercial airliner is descending, just going slowly down, and someone announces, " . . . where the local time *is*—" Well, that's nice to know, to be able to set your watch to the right time, but after that I invariably conveniently forget it. Many things *aren't worth paying attention to anyway*, whether if it's in an airplane descending slowly, or if you're already down there, in that chair. In fact, I've always found it easier to just sit back, let the words drift in, and drift out, and begin to wonder how rapidly I can descend with *one deep breath, or as my rate of breathing changes*, whichever comes first.

restraint

bind of comparable alternatives

A *woman* one time, who was rather deep in a light state of trance, told me that when she wears a digital watch she misses turning the face of the watch toward her and noticing *those hands* out there, because the more she notices them, the second hand moving rather quickly and *lightly*, but sometimes very slowly, and those other two hands, which are either *heavier*, or at least made to move very slowly by comparison. She said that as she notices all those things, she comes to appreciate the definite differences she can invariably and unavoidably oberve in *those hands*.

metaphor

dissociation

ideosensory feeling

dissociation

Bell towers mark time, chiming every so often, sometimes *close by*, sometimes in the *distance*, a sound that tends to drift in and drift out of your hearing, but for lots of people the memory of the sound is stored *in there*, like many other *experiences that can be retrieved when the time is right*. In

apposition of opposites

suggestion

implication

London they have Big Ben, which I've only heard in the movies, never in person, but I can still bring back the face of the clock and its sound.

Someone told me once about an elementary school in a small town in upper Michigan. It was called the Barr school—*two R's in it*—an old red brick, *fluff* two-story building. The man said he had attended the Barr School as well as his mother before him, way back in time. The school's *big bell*, up there in *fluff* the bell tower, you could set your watch by it, and it could be heard from quite a distance, and if you were near the school when that bell rang, like out on the playground, you could actually feel it ring in your body.

Anyway, the Barr School, being very old, *was eventually torn down*. The school's bell was placed near the entrance to the town's historical society, *a modest little building* out by the *fluff* old lighthouse. One day that man, now up in age, and his mother, visited the *historical society building* and on the way in they pulled the rope that rang the bell. Interestingly, the man and his mother, who normally see most things quite differently, both agreed that the sound of the old Barr School bell was exactly the same as they remembered it. The man even indicated that the sound of the bell, in his head, and in his body, *brought back to him some things he had simply forgotten all* about. . . . *suggestion*

After all, a person's *unconscious mind* is a repository of many things: experi- *seeding* ences, memories, resources, perhaps things long forgotten, things that can help you now when you need it the most, so many useful and helpful things in there, deep inside. . . .

Deepening

That's the way, (client's name), doing just fine, breathing comfortably, breathing relaxed, knowing that you can let yourself go just as deep as you desire. Today is Tuesday (or whatever day it is) and you may remember what you had for breakfast this morning, and for dinner last night. But it might be difficult to remember what you had for breakfast—or dinner—Tuesday morning and Monday evening one year ago. Wednesday always comes before Thursday, April always comes before May, always has and always will, and certainly you can remember many things from the past, important things, insignificant things, stored away deep inside.

Everyone enjoys sleeping, and sometimes when you sleep you dream. Maybe you dreamed last night, or early in the morning, and maybe tomorrow you'll have the same dream, or maybe Saturday, like Thursday . . . or maybe next week, but whether this week or next, it really doesn't make any difference.

I know that when I hear a certain song on the radio I'm immediately transported back there, to that time when I heard the song earlier. Now in a moment, (client's name), I'm going to ask you to go back in time, in your mind, to a time, any time at all, when you felt deeply and comfortably relaxed. I don't know if that's yesterday, or six months ago, or ten years ago or more . . . but I'd like you to let your unconscious mind take you back in time, without any conscious effort, going back in time at your own pace and in your own way, to any time at all when you felt deeply and comfortably relaxed . . . and do that now . . . and when you're there, let me know by nodding your head . . . very good.

Pay close attention to yourself back there . . . how old you are . . . whether it's daytime or nightime . . . if you're alone or with others . . . perhaps it's almost as if you're watching on a movie screen, I don't know . . . or maybe you're right up close, or maybe observing at a distance. It really doesn't matter. . . . Just notice the details . . . and let yourself become more and more absorbed in that experience . . . the experience of yourself deeply and comfortably relaxed back then. . . .

REALERTING

Following any additional therapeutic work, the client is asked to return to the present time, and may be alerted by counting from one to five.

DEBRIEFING

In addition to trance-ratifying questions directed at time distortion and ideosensory feelings, open-ended questions such as "How do you feel?" or "What came to mind?" often produce vivid recollections. Pay special attention to the age-regression experience, which can be used for deepening or therapy portions in future sessions.

NOTES FOR PRACTICE

What if you did not receive a discernible head nod when you asked for it during the deepening? This occasionally happens with a permissive suggestion for age regression, but is more common with a directive, authoritarian suggestion such as "I want you to drift back in time now on a magic carpet (or through a time tunnel, or with some other device provided by the therapist) to age ten" (or "before age 30," etc.). By respectfully keeping our suggestions general and permissive, we allow clients to use their imaginations to fill in the blanks, and we are less likely to encounter anxiety or resistance. However, if a head nod is not forthcoming after a minute or two, simply offer a general pacing statement such as, " . . . and anything that is occurring in there is just fine. . . ." This would be a good time to revert to a conventional deepening such as "And now I'm going to count from ten to one, and as I do so, I would like you to imagine youself going deeper and deeper into relaxation." You should never convey to clients that somehow they have failed.

At this point some clients will age regress as initially suggested. Perhaps they feel freed up to do so once the demand has been removed. These things can be discussed—and problem-solved—in the debriefing. As you learn what works for each individual, both induction and deepening can be tailored accordingly.

A majority of clients appear to respond favorably to embedded meaning inductions along with a deepening, such as age regression, that draws on their own experience. Many therapists, having worked with victims of abuse, opt for a "safe place" image either in age regression or as part of a relaxation schema. "Safe place" is an over-used term, and it may carry negative connotations for someone who is not being treated specifically for abuse. In other words, "safe place" for some clients may imply that either something in their history is dangerous or the current therapy setting is unsafe. We prefer expressions like "a time when you felt deeply relaxed." This is more neutral and general.

As with finger signals, sometimes you will not receive a head nod after asking for one. However, during debriefing the client may say, "Oh, I *thought* I nodded my head." If you encounter the same problem in the next session, it may be best to ask for a verbal report. Remember that if past communication in trance has been nonverbal, you cannot just say, "Tell me when you arrive at a time in the past," because clients will think they have to respond nonverbally. People tend to think very concretely in trance; if you want a verbal report you must be very specific, e.g., "When you arrive at a time in the past, tell me *with your words*. . . ."

Subjectively, many clients feel that any overt behavior (head nod, finger signal, or verbal report) will lighten their trance. Accordingly, we always inform clients ahead of time that they will be asked to communicate in one of these ways. Even so, some clients—perhaps ones who want to relax and not really *do* anything—become irritated, especially when we ask them to speak aloud. Others may simply be surprised, having forgotten what we told them, or resent having their trance lightened. Whichever is the case, it may be helpful to suggest, for example, "You may stay deep in trance even while you are speaking," or, if you can discern that trance has indeed lightened, ask them to "Take two deep breaths now . . . and as you exhale that second breath you can feel yourself once again drifting deep into trance, perhaps even deeper than you were before. . . ."

What if the client coughs during any portion of trancework? This happens occasionally and may occur for any number of reasons. Cigarette smokers and people with lung problems may cough frequently. If clients cough recurrently, it is disruptive not only to them, but also to the therapist. We may try normalizing the cough, e.g., ". . . anything that you experience during trance is okay . . . " or utilizing it, ". . . an occasional cough or similar experience may indicate that you are about to relax even more deeply. . . ." However, these measures will be insufficient in the wake of a persistent cough. You may just have to stop the process and try again next session. Certainly, a cough is every bit a challenge to the therapist as pain, hearing loss, and unconscious resistance. A cough drop, a drink of water, a dose of inhaler medication (if they have it with them), or a positional shift (lying down or sitting up) may help.

GOING INSIDE

We have all worked with clients who want to be told what to do. Sometimes we oblige them, but more often we help them to generate their own solutions. The client who is very concrete, personality disordered, or of low intelligence can be even more challenging. With these populations, it may be necessary to help clients recognize appropriate changes.

We often use the following induction and deepening in order to stimulate an internal search for resources. How do we know if we are successful? Clients may show concomitant improvement on a self-efficacy or depression scale; objectively, they may seem to have improved. Although we seek to generate new behavior, a demonstration of new internal resources may be very modest in people who lead rather marginal lives. It may be something like "I decided to go back to Alcoholics Anonymous" or, "I started back to church" or even, "I've been thinking more about things." After this induction one client stated that he began watching the cartoon channel, whereas previously he had preferred the weather channel. For him, this represented a veritable paradigm shift, and soon he demonstrated a whole range of new behavior.

The deepening with this induction involves an often-told story about Milton Erickson. People with disabilities or fractured lives seem to enjoy stories about this famous wounded healer who, like many of them, came from another state before settling in Arizona. In pre-trance discussion we talk about Erickson, who survived polio as a youth and endured great pain and disability during his life.

As with other inductions in which the goal is unconscious stimulation or search, clients may need a concrete description of the unconscious mind, e.g., "the part of your mind that takes over when you dream—or daydream." Also, the word "imagination" may capture the concept for them. Suggestions and hypnotic concepts that are highlighted may be read with a change in your voice.

Induction

Jacquelyn Burns was lost in deep thought as she gazed out the window of her executive suite on the 46th floor. Her boss's words still rang in her head. *"Go inside*, Burns." When she asked for an explanation, all he said was, *"Go inside*. You figure it out."

Jacquelyn Burns headed up the advertising company's division, which included 19 major accounts for toothpaste, rental cars, and hardware stores. In her years with the company, she recognized that change was inevitable and that things can happen for different reasons. She had rolled with the punches and her creativity and drive had propelled her to the top in her field.

Jacquelyn assembled a task force of subordinates and gave them their assignment. "We need to *go inside*," she said.

"What do you mean by *'go inside'*?" they asked.

"You figure it out. We need to *go inside*. Report back to me in thirty days," she directed.

After much discussion and brainstorming, the rental car division task force implemented the following plan. They got approval from authorities to install videocameras at the entrance to a busy freeway, at a stop light, and at the detour on a less traveled city street. Remote viewing rooms were set up at several locations and people were hired to record their observations during morning and afternoon rush hour.

"I still wonder what Burns *really* means when she says, *'go inside*,'" said one of the people in the task force, as she opened up a file in the computer. Another woman, who wadded up a piece of paper and lazily suspended it over the wastebasket before dropping it in, commented, "They say it came down from the top, but I say this *inside* stuff came from the outside." A third woman, observing from across the room, felt compelled to answer both observations about this new *inside* turn of events, but she chose to just mull it over in her own mind for the time being.

Task force workers at the remote viewing locations witnessed many things. Some drivers were observed with their windows open, even when the temperature was above 100 degrees. Drivers of two Wal-Mart trucks both looked bored, and the driver of a school bus talked in animated fashion to children over her shoulder, while the driver of another school bus seemed oblivious to anything but his own deep thought. Drivers and passengers in RVs looked straight ahead while waiting for the light to change, and in a Lincoln Continental—with the windows up—two retired men sat in the front seat while in the back two women with gray hair and straw hats carried on a spirited conversation. Teenage drivers in several vehicles kept time to music on the radio, totally unaware of cars in front and cars in back. People in vans that were obvious car pools appeared to be engaged in conversation more in the afternoon than in the morning, but then again, the opposite proved to be true at other times.

Now it happened that people in the remote viewing locations *began to let their own minds wander* as they observed what went on *inside* all those vehicles. They thought about their own driving experiences, how they *easily became bored* with driving down the road, and how looking up ahead on a winding road it was difficult to tell on which side of the road sat the convenience store, but how *at the same time it really didn't matter* as they would find out when they got there.

Some people watching became *fascinated* with the *curious* activity of the thousands of drivers they observed, while others became *immersed in anything* but the job at hand, while still others *became absorbed in* their own reflections on many things. Some thought about their own thoughts while being stuck in traffic, as well as their own frustration or impatience with the *slowness of the road*. Others ruminated or inwardly examined innumerable things that were seemingly unrelated to anything. One woman thought, "Looking from in here out there at all the activity inside those vehicles is *one of the stranger detachments that I have ever experienced*."

Certainly it was impolite to stare too long at someone in the lane next to them, and you could look longer at someone in one of the side mirrors, but in the rearview mirror lengthy glances could become very obvious. One person *noticed* a woman handing her child a Kleenex and, as he watched her *hand suspended in the air*, he couldn't help but reflect on his own similar experience not too long ago. As he remembered it—and of course, a person's memory of anything can become fuzzy over time—he *could not recall* if he had held that Kleenex out for mere seconds, or if the *blurring of time* had simply caused a minute to seem like an hour.

A blue haze of cigar smoke swirled inside the cab of a furniture store delivery truck and more than one person watching this coughed reflexively. Another person watched a lowrider quiver with the boom of loud music and she responded viscerally, a churning in her stomach and a reverberation in her ears, or was it inside her head? Another person *noticed* a driver with his arm draped across the top of the seat. Having his arm in that position for several minutes at the detour reminded one observer of her own arm *after she had slept on it* at night. Certainly to *lose feeling* in something like an arm—or a hand—cannot be much different than a shot of novacaine from the dentist, she thought.

These observations and reflections went on for several weeks as the behavior of thousands of drivers was scrutinized and duly recorded. Finally the head of the task force announced, "Our job is done. I believe that we have successfully captured both the letter and the spirit of our assignment." When Jacquelyn Burns read the report, she was *pleasantly surprised*, and she knew her boss would be, too.

However, with the passage of time, some of the people who had staffed the remote viewing locations missed their job. As they worked on other assignments much different from this one, their *minds drifted once again* as they fondly contemplated the experience.

Deepening

(Client's name), listening to this story, some thoughts or feelings or ideas may have come to you. In a moment I'm going to tell you another little story, a story about Dr. Erickson that I mentioned earlier, and while you listen to this story, I would like you to *go inside even more deeply*, and we know that this can happen all by itself, without any conscious effort on your part. . . . Take two more deep, deep breaths now, and just let yourself drift, that's right. . . .

Some years ago Dr. Erickson was giving some lectures in the Midwest. It may have been Milwaukee, I forget for sure, and when he was there someone asked him to visit a depressed woman who would not leave her house. The woman formerly attended her church where she had many friends, but she had not seen any of them for a long, long time. Being a very curious and helpful man, Dr. Erickson gladly *looked in* on what sounded like a most interesting situation.

Once *inside*, he noticed that the house was very dark, even though it was the middle of the day. He asked the woman to show him around the house. It was a big, three-story house with many rooms, and Dr. Erickson insisted on visiting every room, and from inside every room he could see that the curtains were drawn, keeping out the light of day. Dr. Erickson was keenly observant with the front part of his mind, while the back part of his mind surveyed many things, and way back in the house, up on the third floor he noticed *light coming in* through one small window, and on a small table in front of the window was a flower pot with beautiful African violets. The woman perked up a bit as she commented proudly about her violets. "Hmmm," responded Dr. Erickson as they continued their tour through the big, dark house.

Dr. Erickson said nothing else to the woman until he bid her farewell at the front door. Then he casually added, "Wouldn't it be nice if people in your church could enjoy those wonderful African violets?" Then he left and he never saw the woman again.

Months later, someone reported to Dr. Erickson that the woman was feeling much better and was regularly attending church. It turns out that, as she started to grow more and more violets, she had to open the curtains in room after room, *letting in the light,* and because so many people in town enjoyed her violets she became known as the African violet queen.

REALERTING

As our goal is unconscious acceptance of the African violets story, we realert with the following: "In a moment I will ask you to reawaken, but first, I want to ask a question of your unconscious mind, and you may answer with one of those fingers on your right hand. The question is this: The story about Dr. Erickson, is that something that you are willing to contemplate between now and the next time you return here? Taking as much time as you need, you may answer with a finger signal . . . very good.

"Now I'd like you to reawaken at your own pace and open your eyes."

DEBRIEFING

Some clients may respond to the implicit demand of this induction and deepening by saying, "This made me think of such-and-such," but we quickly end discussion with "Let's let your unconscious mind work on this for a while, and I'll ask you next time what has come up." Also, it is always helpful to ratify trance as previously outlined.

NOTES FOR PRACTICE

Bright, imaginative, and highly motivated clients may progress rapidly in therapy. However, with concrete or unsophisticated clients, we may need to go more slowly. Generating resources or making an unconscious commitment may be far removed from their everyday experience. Accordingly, it may be better to alternate a session such as the above with a conversational induction and deepening for the purpose of relaxation. We should plan where we want clients to go, but if they are overwhelmed by too much too quickly, they might not return. In fact, we do not advocate hypnosis in every session with any client. Sometimes it is necessary to deal with something, such as a crisis, that must be processed verbally. Other times, a behavioral or related application may be the best use of therapy time. Generally, it is a good idea to periodically take stock of where the therapy is going, and this must be communicated orally.

When a client has responded with finger signals in previous sessions and suddenly ceases to do so, consider buttressing the suggestion with metaphor in order to free up a response. For example, if we ask an unconsciously-directed question and no finger movement occurs after a minute or two, then we might say, "One time someone imagined a balloon up at the ceiling and a string from the balloon lifted up just one finger down below. . . ." or, "I had a bucket of water and a large cork, and I held the cork under the water and when I let it go it just popped up to the surface. . . ." or, "One time I was at a musical performance. Up on the stage they stopped playing, and after an awkward silence one person clapped, and then applause just rippled through the audience. . . ." However, with clients we do not know well, we usually refrain from such examples. We do not want to pressure them or to contribute to any power struggle.

SLOWING DOWN

Anxiety and stress management are often presenting problems, so naturally we look for different ways to help our clients *slow down*. Some clients with generalized anxiety disorder or anxiety secondary to another diagnosis may benefit immensely from a few sessions of hypnotherapy. These clients are likely to respond to any number of inductions such as those found in this book. Installing an anchor, such as a deep breath, and giving clients an individualized audiotape may help them manage their anxiety for some time.

For other clients who present with anxiety, we may discuss reordering priorities, better time management, or merely simplifying a busy life. However, many people have already attempted to use these concrete measures before they sought help. Some have tried yoga, meditation, prayer, self-help tapes, conventional psychotherapy, and even hypnotherapy before we see them. In other words, clients know where they want to go, but they cannot get started. "Something is holding me back," they may say, or "Medication helps—but it only helps so much."

Let's assume that such a person functions fairly well in life and scores unremarkably on a depression or anxiety scale. In the past we may have labeled this person neurotic or laden with angst, typical of the "healthy but unhappy" client we might see in our practice. He seeks the ability to *slow down* and enjoy some peace in this busy electronic world, but he cannot get started, and cannot *get from here to there*. *Something* is holding him back, blocking the way, or weighing him down. We could work for months, or even years, in talk therapy, exploring this elusive *something*.

Or, we can *indirectly* engage this "traveler who has yet to arrive" by simply bypassing this *something*. We see this clinical presentation in the same light as the unconscious resistance evinced by people who *want* to go into trance, but cannot: *something* is holding them back. Catalepsy is the hypnotic phenomenon at play in these situations, so movement may need to be suggested. Such movement does not necessarily imply speed, but rather an absence of inertia. We believe that one of the major benefits of an indirect hypnotherapeutic approach is that it accesses unconscious resources, freeing people to put change into motion. Such movement could include behavioral activation, new learning, a different way of thinking or feeling about something, or some other novel experience.

One of the principal ways we begin to access unconscious resources is through inductions driven by embedded meaning. As many clients are unaccustomed to indirection, they may need to be trained, both by pre-trance discussion about the unconscious mind as well as by experience in trance. Experience in trance could mean a series of inductions (such as Embedded Meaning) that stimulate the imagination, or therapeutic stories, which connect with clients emotionally, allowing important learning to be integrated into their cognitive structure. As with the other inductions, "woman" can be substituted for "man" and italicized words may be given vocal emphasis. Seeding *"slowing down"* in pre-trance discussion sets up this induction, which should be reeled out *slowly* with ample pauses.

Induction

Not too long ago a woman was telling me her various experiences with *slowing down*.

At first I wasn't sure what she was talking about, but it became clear after a short time. She spoke rather *slowly* which was good because I paid careful attention to the words, noticing many details and appreciating her special understanding of *slowing down* in everyday experience. She mentioned time as told by an hourglass and contrasted this with time on a clock with hands. She knew full well that some children these days can't tell time on anything other than a digital clock.

When she sat very still she could really notice the feel of her clothes as well as other interesting sensations like the prickliness in her scalp or a tingling sensation in her body. At a shopping mall one time she sat down, just sat there very still and tuned out all the noise. She sat for what seemed like a long, long time, although in reality not much time had passed at all, people streaming by, just a blur of movement. All of a sudden someone passed by very *slowly*, which definitely arrested attention. That person who took so long to walk by reminded her of other pattern interruptions, when you are observing something, or doing something, over and over and over again and unexpectedly *something different* catches our attention.

All the while she talked about things going on *outside*, she began to *slow down* on the *inside*, and she called this both a comfortable and interesting experience, not unlike something she had done some time in the past, but she couldn't remember exactly when.

She said that a tree grows rather *slowly*, but with flowers and other plants you can see changes week to week. She remembered once seeing the morning sun shine pink through a rabbit's ear, and the smell of chalk dust brought back memories of her schoolroom long ago. It was interesting how these and other memories lingered *slowly* in her mind. "Delicately *delayed*," she termed it.

Talking about memories allowed her to appreciate *slowing down* on the inside while describing outside phenomena, and this produced a similar *slowing down*, "a *slowness deeper* inside" was the way she put it. "It developed *deeper* in a *slow* and gradual sort of way," she added, along with something about the "growth of a strong tree, its branches up above and roots deep down below," but I forget exactly what the words were way back then.

She remembered once how they built a skyscraper and *down* in the bottom they sealed up a time capsule, which someone would find someday. Years passed and then one day she found herself walking by that building. It was a warm, sunny day. As she talked about this she was unaware of curling up her toes *inside* her shoes, and she continued to talk about time capsules and even the idea of time travel as it is depicted in science fiction.

On a plane one time she flew through several time zones. In a big country like Russia with nine time zones people would probably forget to keep setting their watches, but doing so *really wouldn't matter* until you got where you were going. The idea of time zones produced a different sort of *slowing down* inside both her mind and her body, though the feeling wasn't really connected. "Together but at the same time apart" was her description. I knew what she meant by that. Her *hands felt heavy* out there on her lap.

She recalled how the evening before bedtime often passes rather quickly and time on a vacation is seldom *slow*. While out there driving, a person waits for a light to change, which is invariably *slow*, as is time sitting in a meeting or a class. She thought about how quickly something came to mind once and how then her mind *lingered* on just why that thought had occurred precisely then. Was it a word or something else that stimulated the experience of having been there some time before? Perhaps it was yesterday or many years before, she would never know. At any rate, by thinking about all these things, her mind had suddenly become very active while her body had really *slowed down* by comparison.

Deepening

Now, as I count down from 20 to one, I would like you to notice which one of the following applies in your case: whether the numbers counted backward are fast or *slow*. Or whether the pace picks up after an even number right before an odd number. Or whether *slowness* fills the space between all the numbers. Or whether you can relate any slowness in general to slowing down in your mind, or your body, in particular.

The important thing to remember is that I'm going to count *very, very slowly* from 20 to one, and during this time you can let your experience deepen. Beginning to count now, 20 . . . , 19 . . . .

REALERTING

With the clinical presentation described above, we may not include a therapy component. We realert accordingly: "(Client's name), today you did a commendable job—and made a major effort—just imagining *slowing down*, which we all know can be a very good thing. Now I want you to quickly draw a contrast to this experience by waking up *very fast* as I count from one to five. One-two-three-four-five."

DEBRIEFING

Listen very closely to the client's first few sentences coming out of trance. Things said at this time may be gifts they bestow unknowingly, things that can be utilized next time. For example, one client said, "I was having these visual fireworks—it was fabulous." A somewhat oppositional client remarked, "In my head I counted from 20 to one *fast*, and I got there long before you did!" The client with the visual fireworks provided a useful touchstone that eventually permitted the induction to be shortened to a few deep breaths and "letting yourself drift deeply into relaxation, and taking as much time as you need, when you can imagine those visual fireworks, let me know with your *yes* finger."

The fast counter's offering was utilized by reframing the behavior as eagerness and responsibility in not dissipating valuable time. I (GG) asked her to teach me this ability to go deep swiftly by doing it ten times in succession after the induction. This client did quite nicely in therapy afterward, and I'm sure she never realized just how much she taught me about utilization.

NOTES FOR PRACTICE

Although embedded meaning drives this induction, the multiple bind deepening and the fast realerting add confusional elements.

With clients for whom your goal is to bypass unconscious resistance, we recommend trying this induction, deepening, and realerting. The meta-message (*slowing down*) is more likely to be accepted. Some clients will respond to this type of induction with deep trance, especially characterized by time distortion, amnesia, and a dazed countenance when realerted. These clients are likely to respond well to a less confusional induction next time, e.g., the road, travel induction, or any of the conversational inductions in Chapter 2. In other words, you have successfully countered their unwitting resistance; now they are ready for finger signals and other aspects of therapy. Many of these clients do well with continued indirection and inducing amnesia for an anecdote or story. Inducing amnesia allows the unconscious to work on the problem without conscious interference. This may be very helpful with resistant or extremely analytical clients. See the Going Inside and Erickson Meets Huxley inductions for further discussion of these techniques.

This induction also works well without the confusional elements. For example, in an anxiety problem not complicated by resistance, the Slowing Down induction is useful with a standard deepening. We have also used it as an ego-strengthening story in therapy, because skill building and gaining mastery can definitely boost one's self-efficacy.

ERICKSON MEETS HUXLEY

We devised this induction for a 75-year-old client, a retired mathematics professor with a rather sophisticated knowledge of both psychotherapy and hypnotherapy. As a 17-year-old soldier, he was among the first ashore at Omaha Beach in the invasion of Normandy during World War II. However, prolonged exposure to combat had caused no PTSD symptoms and he functioned quite well throughout his life. This man, whom we will call Sam, was diagnosed with dysthymia, although he believed himself to be profoundly and incurably depressed. Through the years, Sam had tried a panoply of medications and therapeutic modalities without success. He had read about Milton Erickson and was eager to try Ericksonian hypnotherapy, although he wasn't really sure what that meant. We had unsuccessfully attempted conversational inductions with him, along with interventions directed at altering his monolithic, self-defeating views.

Sam enjoyed reading; he had read Aldous Huxley. Also, he prized his daily walks as a time when "I can clear my head." As an induction, we adapted a published account of Erickson's meeting Huxley (Rossi, 1980), and fashioned two alternating stories, devised by colleagues Dr. Matt Weyer and Dr. Julie Feldman, as a deepening. The embedded meaning (walk and move) in the deepening is true embedded meaning, while the various suggestions of hypnotic phenomena in the induction are more by proxy, much like the My Friend John induction (Chapter 6). In the pre-trance discussion with Sam we amply seeded *walk* and *move*, and, to distract his busy mind, we asked him to count the number of times he heard the word *trance* during the induction. Hypnotic phenomena or key concepts are italicized and should be read with a subtle emphasis.

Sam sat back and closed his eyes without being asked to do so, and thus we began.

Induction

Early in 1950, Phoenix psychiatrist Milton Erickson drove to Los Angeles to meet with the famous British writer, Aldous Huxley. In those days the drive took a bit longer, and going down the road Erickson's mind *wandered*, as it was prone to do, and he *wondered* about Huxley. The two did not know each other and were from very different backgrounds; nevertheless, they had heard of each other and they agreed to meet for a joint inquiry into various states of psychological awareness. Although Huxley had no formal training in hypnosis, he was known for his own unique use of the *unconscious mind* as well as his ability as a subject to demonstrate a *deep somnambulistic trance*.

Erickson's interest in this joint venture had to do with psychological experimentation, while Huxley had in mind future literary work. In fact, in 1954 he published his famous work, *Doors of Perception*. During their meetings, which lasted 10 hours each day, both men recorded their observations in several loose-leaf notebooks. The notebooks were left with Huxley at the conclusion of the meetings. Shortly thereafter, a brushfire destroyed Huxley's home and all its contents, including the loose-leaf notebooks. The project was never discussed again and was seemingly forgotten until years later when Erickson discovered separate notes that he had made of his encounter with Huxley.

As he looked over his notes, Erickson remembered how Huxley described a *light trance state* in which he experienced "a simple *withdrawal of interest from the outside to the inside*" during which time there persisted a *"dim but ready" awareness* that he could alter a state of awareness at will. He contrasted this with a *medium trance*, which he termed a "most pleasing subjective sense of *comfort*" and "a vague, *dim awareness* that there was an external reality." If he examined an item of external reality—for example, the *feeling of the chair beneath him,* or the quiet of the room, he invariably went deeper into trance.

Huxley was eager to discuss what he called a state of *deep reflection*. Huxley said he could enter a state of *deep reflection* in about five minutes. "I simply cast off all anchors," he stated. This was marked by a state of physical *relaxation*, closed eyes, a *turning inward*, and a profound, progressive *psychological withdrawal* from the external world. It was a "setting aside" of everything not pertinent and a state of *complete mental absorption* in matters of interest to him. Physical activity did not slow or impede his train of thought, and everything going on outside himself seemed like *completely peripheral activity*. "I might say activity *barely contiguous to the periphery*," Huxley added. He cited as an example how he would be in a state of *deep reflection* while working on a manuscript. The phone would ring and he would write down the message for his wife, but later when his wife came home he had *no memory* of either the phone call or the note.

One day Erickson and Huxley performed an experiment. Before *entering the state*, Erickson asked Huxley if he would later awaken when he heard three taps of a pencil on the table. Huxley quickly went *into trance* and during the next several minutes Erickson tapped the pencil four times in succession, two times, eight times, using different variations and intervals, and Huxley did not respond. Erickson even tipped over a chair loudly onto the floor, and Huxley remained in *deep reflection*. Finally, Erickson tapped three times, and Huxley awakened, *totally unaware* of what had happened. He reported only a vague sensation "that something was coming," but he knew not what. Huxley had *absolutely no awareness* of what had been done.

Another time Erickson induced a trance and Huxley reported afterward that he had *"lost"* himself in a "sea of color, of *being* . . . *sensing* . . . and *feeling* quite utterly involved with no identity of my own." Quite suddenly, he experienced a process of losing that color in a "meaningless void," only to open his eyes and realize he had "come out of it." Huxley repeatedly commented on his experience in trance: " . . . utterly amazing . . . most extraordinary. . . ."

Huxley also wished to experiment with different levels of trance. In a *light trance*, Huxley found himself "drifting along . . . with a 'dim but ready' awareness that he could alter his state of awareness at will, or that he could 'reach out and seize external reality'." In a *medium trance*, Huxley found that he had a subjective need to go *deeper into trance*, and that he had an intellectual need to stay at a *medium level of trance*. Once in a *medium trance*, he found that when he examined an item of external reality for subjective value—for example, the soft comfort of the chair cushions as contrasted to the intrinsic quiet of the room—the trance became *deeper*.

Erickson and Huxley then wondered about developing hallucinatory phenomena *in both light and medium trances*. While Huxley had hallucinations of taste, he was unaware that his *swallowing increased* while he did this. Similarly, when he experienced hallucinations of smell, his *nostrils flared*, again, without realizing that he was doing so. They eventually progressed to both auditory and visual hallucinations, during which time Huxley heard music and saw a giant rose, perhaps three feet in diameter. About this time he smelled something very bad, and he described the experience as "intense . . . distinctly unroselike," *truly a most curious experience*.

They eventually progressed to super memory, difficult to test in Huxley's case because of his extreme capacity to recall past events. While Huxley was in both *light and medium trances*, Erickson took a random book off the shelf, read a few words from a page, and with 65-percent accuracy Huxley could recite the remainder of the paragraph and tell the page number in the book.

They then experimented with Huxley's being in a *deep somnambulistic trance* in which he experienced a peculiar *restriction of awareness* where everything was very literal and concrete. For example, when he opened his eyes during trance he could see only things very close to him, the chair on which he sat, and Erickson's chair, right there in front of him.

Erickson's notes as well as his recollection of the experience ended there. For years afterward he thought about Huxley's capability of *deep reflection*.

Deepening

Now, (client's name), I would like you to cease counting the word "trance" and just let your experience deepen while I tell you a couple of little stories. Someone told me once about a man named Bruce, the best cook he ever knew. Bruce went to different schools to be a chef, and he even worked at several fine restaurants, but he never quite cooked up to his potential. But things began to change for him one day when he found something. To his great surprise, way back in the cupboard among the various pots and pans, he found his old *wok*.

At about the same time, on the west coast, there was a woman named Alison who was very adept in many areas of her life. To remain successful she had *moved* around quite a bit . . . and as you may know, *moving* is no easy endeavor, especially when you have other people to consider. And now it was time to *move* once again.

That *wok* was covered with rust and had not been used for many years. He remembered the trouble he always had with Asian dishes, but at the same time his classmates at chef school had become quite adept at *woking*. "You notice a lot of things about cooking when you get lost in *woking*," they had told him.

Back on the west coast, Alison had selected a *moving* company, and she chose to follow the *moving* truck across the country, up and down the hills, across the plains, and at times it seemed like a very directionless affair, even though she found herself *moved* considerably by the natural beauty that a person comes to appreciate going across the United States.

In his kitchen Bruce began to experiment with his *wok*, first with one kind of oil, and then another; and first on low heat, then on medium heat, and eventually on high heat. He did a lot of thinking when he worked with his *wok*, but mostly he contemplated, deep inside, "I can do this, really I can." And little by little he improved, and eventually he got it just right. The Asian dishes he prepared were tantalizing, absolutely marvelous, and employment in five-star restaurants soon followed.

REALERTING

In order to offer a posthypnotic suggestion and facilitate amnesia, we may realert with the following: "(Client's name), you did a commendable job here today, counting, listening, and going into trance, and already I'm beginning to wonder, (client's name), just wonder, between now and the next time you return, *what important thing about yourself will you notice when you're outside*? In a moment I'm going to count from one up to five, at which time you can reawaken, but first, let me ask you to conveniently forget anything you may have intended to remember, and beginning to count now one, two, *four* . . . and five."

DEBRIEFING

When clients open their eyes, they often appear disoriented. When you ask them what they remember, some say, "Erickson . . . Huxley . . . something about a moving company. . . ." Other clients will be amnesic to all content.

NOTES FOR PRACTICE

In the next session, some clients may report something like "I realized I need to make some changes." A few will be able to connect this realization to an activity, such as taking a walk. Many will make no such connection, because the suggestion during the realerting ("notice something important about yourself when you are outside") is "forgotten" to allow the unconscious to solve the problem without conscious interference. It is more likely to be effective if you tag the suggestion to a naturally occurring behavior, such as walking. Amnesia is seeded in the induction and activated in the realerting with both a direct suggestion to forget as well as the omission of the number three in counting up. A person's attention is drawn to something that is obviously missing, which consequently facilitates amnesia (Jefferey Zeig, personal communication, 1998). Deep trance is usually necessary for this to be successful.

Clients who respond well to this approach will usually do well with a conversational induction and standard counting-down deepening for the remainder of therapy. We would customarily continue indirection by first installing ideomotor finger signals, and then telling an ego-strengthening story as part of therapy. Following the story, clients are asked, "Is this something that your unconscious mind can put to use? You may answer with one of your fingers." If the I-don't-know/I-don't-want-to-answer-yet finger raises, we would follow with this question: "Is this something your unconscious mind is willing to think about between now and next time?" Most often they will answer the question with a yes finger. Thereafter clients often answer affirmatively when asked the first question.

Whatever happened to our client Sam? After five sessions of hypnotherapy he said he felt better and he no longer evinced his former angst and negativity. He declined a referral for either standard cognitive therapy or group therapy, explaining that he would prefer to just keep taking his long daily walks. We never heard from Sam again, and we can only hope that he continues walking for a long, long time.

RAINMAKER

In some of the inductions in this book we mention hypnotic language, words such as "imagine" and "curious," that are believed to stimulate a sense of wonderment or hypnoid behavior. One of the most potent words in this category may be "story." When we say to clients, "Let me tell you a little story," they immediately begin to focus on the words that follow. Story is both an ancient tradition and a universal experience. Clients were undoubtedly told stories as children, and the tradition likely continues into their present experience in a variety of ways. They may read stories to themselves, their children, or grandchildren, or they may encounter stories in movies, songs, or religious tradition.

Sometimes we induce trance simply by telling a story. The story need not have embedded suggestions for any trance phenomena. Clients' attention becomes absorbed while listening, and, as absorption occurs, they become receptive to the meta-meaning or metaphor inherent in the story. Many times we offer clients vague stories whose metaphor could be interpreted in numerous ways. We never explain what the story is intended to convey, but instead ask them to "let it rest in your unconscious mind for a while before you jump to any conclusions."

A while back I (SB) had a client we'll call Hiram, a man in his fifties who was moderately overweight. He had tried many things to lose weight, and now he was asking for hypnosis. What impressed me most about Hiram in the initial interview was that he appeared *ready* to change. The problem, accordingly to him, was "I have no willpower." When he returned, I told him a story we call "The Rainmaker," and, as a deepening, offered him an embedded-meaning story that addressed his presenting problem. Thanks to Dr. Bob Hall for "The Rainmaker."

Induction

I've heard this story many times, and each time I hear it I wonder about the meaning it has, if any. Some people have said, "It means *this*," and others have said, "It means *that*," and still others have said that it means nothing at all. However, I like the story just the same, and I will tell it to you now. It's called "The Rainmaker."

Years ago, in some distant land across the sea, a village of people had endured months of drought, and there was no sign of rain any time soon. Many feared that they would lose their crops, and there was much worry and tension in the village.

One day a wise old man who was known far and wide as the Rainmaker appeared in the village. His words to the head of the village were few: "Build me a hut and leave me alone in there for three full days." A hut was readily assembled and the Rainmaker entered.

One day passed and still there was no sign of rain. By the end of the second day the sky remained clear. People in the village began to worry more than ever. Some paced in the sand in front of the Rainmaker's hut, some wrung their hands and pulled their hair. One man even tore his loin cloth in desperation, but most villagers just worried in silence.

By the middle of the third day there still was no sign of rain. Tension ran high. One man said he dreamed of vultures the night before. Mothers clutched their children, and there was moaning and tears among the elders. Late that afternoon dark clouds began to fill the sky, and shortly afterward the rain poured down.

As the people rejoiced, the Rainmaker slowly emerged from his hut. The villagers rushed to his side, threw themselves at his feet, and thanked him profusely for all he had done. The Rainmaker rubbed sleep from his eyes and a puzzled look appeared on his face. Finally he said, "But I haven't done anything yet. I was ill and needed to rest for three days."

Deepening

I would like you to let your experience deepen as I tell you another story. Someone I know named Angela was telling me just the other day about her mother, who lives down the road in Tucson. Her mother lives next to TEP—that stands for Tucson Electric Power. One day her mom was out for her daily walk and she met a man who worked at TEP. It was late in the afternoon and it was a very hot day. It turned out the man's name was *Will*, *Will* from the *power* plant, who was outside enjoying a light lunch. Well, Angela's mother, being a friendly sort, began a conversation. Her mom is a serious student of meditation and soon she and *Will* were discussing the *power* of the unconscious mind. *Will* agreed that the mind is indeed very *power*ful and he even told a story of his own meditative experience.

One time in trance, *Will* from the *power* plant told her mom, he had an awareness of himself breaking through some of his bad habits. In addition, his strength—both his inner strength and resolve as well as the strength of his body—were brought into his conscious mind. After that *power*ful experience *Will* said he felt more enlightended and had a new resolve to be a more holistically healthy person. Angela's mother, entranced by his story, smiled and said she meditates frequently and was glad to find a kindred spirit. Then she continued on her routine walk, happy to have strengthened a bond with *Will* from the *power* plant.

REALERTING

In fitting with the casual induction, we like to tell clients that the story is completed and that they can return to their alert state.

DEBRIEFING

Similarly casual and general inquiries, such as "What are you thinking?" or "What are you feeling now?" may be made. At this juncture clients will often ask questions such as "What did that story mean?" Of course, we never provide a meaningful answer. Some may experience amnesia for the first story, but let us know that the embedded meaning in the second story was obvious to them. As with the first story, we divert their attention and ask them to let their unconscious mull it over between now and next time.

NOTES FOR PRACTICE

If clients return and are imaginally stimulated by this approach, we will then offer more of the same, activating unconscious resources and helping them find their own solutions to problems. In this way, the therapist is really just a guide who provides the client with a general framework. With these clients we would also set up finger signals and seek unconscious commitment, as discussed in other inductions.

With some clients this casual, general, and permissive approach falls flat. They may evince few indicators of trance, or they may be bored by the process. In such cases we would attempt a conversational or embedded-meaning induction to try to build their response.

And overweight Hiram? He responded well to this induction and deepening. He never mentioned willpower again, nor did I. He was seen three more times before beginning serious participation in a structured weight reduction program with a physician and dietitian.

One of the greatest values of this very nondirective approach is that it helps *set up* the client for needed change. Hiram was ready to change and just needed a nudge. Others may need ego-strengthening, therapeutic stories with unconscious commitment, or simply unconscious search to uncover obstacles to growth. Once these are accomplished, the client is usually ready for further hypnotherapeutic applications or conventional talk therapy.

Story is an exceptionally versatile device in hypnotherapy. It can be a strong, effective part of induction, deepening, or therapy. We employ a story alone, a story within a story, two or more alternating stories, and story without an ending. The story with no ending stimulates an immediate unconscious search whose discovery may be evident next session. Or we may encourage unconscious search in a guided fashion. At the completion of the story (with no ending), we ask the client to provide an ending, e.g., "Taking as much time as you need, when an ending, any kind of ending at all, surfaces from your unconscious mind, your yes finger will twitch and develop a lightness all its own, and move up into the air." We ask for a verbal report following the finger signal. The process can also be repeated. Debriefing may also yield further information.

4

Confusional Inductions

CANDLE FLAME

This induction developed in my (GG) pro bono work with refugees from Central America. Many of these people came from Guatemala and El Salvador, where years of civil war led to the kidnapping, torture, massacre, disappearance, and murder of literally hundreds of thousands of the indigenous population (Melville & Lykes, 1992). In their native land, these clients' lives were filled with fear and persecution. Chronic, severe **PTSD** and major depression complicate their adjustment. Fischman (1991) and Pope and Garcia-Peltoniemi (1991) review the various issues involved in treating the psychological aftereffects of political repression and torture. Acculturation to the United States is a slow process, and for some, Spanish (which I speak) is a second language to their indigenous tongue. Few have any experience with mental health treatment as we know it. However, when referred for mental health treatment, they are usually agreeable participants, perhaps because mental health is an integral part of the medical model at this university family practice clinic. Some of these clients have been started on medication before we see them.

Psychoeducation regarding PTSD is sometimes futile. Even after being provided with explanations complete with illustrations, clients may still believe that they are anxious, for example, "because of the pill they gave me in Guatemala." Nevertheless, they do desire relief from their symptoms, and hypnotherapy is one of the modalities available. This induction has also been used with refugees from Africa, who in many cases experienced even worse torture and cruelty than people from Central America.

I soon learned to forget about suggesting eye closure: few ever wished to do so. These clients readily become absorbed in eye fixation, and I arbitrarily began to use the flame of a Catholic saint candle, which they seemed to like. In addition to the candle flame, I use two alternating inductions to further absorb their attention and, hopefully, make therapeutic gains at the same time. As many of these clients are very somatic, a direct suggestion of warm liquid going down their body is alternated with an ego-strengthening story. As I alternate between the warm liquid metaphor and the ego-strengthening story, *clients themselves count aloud*, slowly, from 100 to one, while remaining absorbed in the candle.

Clients are informed that the therapist will be giving suggestions for bodily relaxation and telling them a story that is directed at the unconscious mind. "The part of your mind that takes over when you are dreaming" conveys the concept to most of these clients. They indicate their agreement to count backward while looking at the flame.

Induction

You may continue to keep your eyes focused on the flame of that candle, and while you are doing that I will continue to talk to you, and those words might drift in and drift out, but you don't have to pay attention to the words, because your unconscious mind can pay especially close attention and help you at this time, that's the way, just

100

99

98

looking at that flame. You don't have to   *97*
do anything else at all, and if your eyes
become tired and want to close, they
may, all by themselves, or else you can   *96*
continue to become pleasantly and
comfortably absorbed in that flame,
breathing in comfort and relaxation,   *95*
that's the way, deep comfortable
breaths, letting your mind and body
become more and more relaxed.   *94*

Now, (client's name), I'd like you to
imagine a warm and pleasant feeling
starting to develop and spread out, up   *93*
there at the top of your head. You can
imagine the feeling of a warm liquid or
something else that is pleasant and   *92*
comfortable, and when you can imag-
ine that, let me know by nodding your
head . . . good, that's the way.   *91*

Now let that comfortable feeling go
all down the back of your head, that's
right. Each part of your body that gets   *90*
touched by that feeling will feel more
and more slowed down and relaxed . . .
and now down your neck, deeply and   *89*
comfortably relaxed.

Every day on his (her) way to school
a young (wo)man walked by this mag-   *88*
nificent greenhouse. He noticed all the
beautiful plants growing in there, dark
green leaves of different sizes and flow-   *87*
ers with bright, lovely colors. One day
he asked if he could work in the greenhouse for the summer, and the boss   *86*
said, "Sure, but it's hard work and you
have to pay close attention to what
you're doing."   *85*

Nice comfortable feeling going all
down your back, down, down your
shoulder blades and down your spine,   *84*

slowly, comfortably, more and more
slowed down and relaxed, feeling
good. . . .   *83*

Now that young man started to work
and he worked very hard every day. He
swept the floor, carried bags of soil and   *82*
peat moss, and moved plants around
the big greenhouse. Every once in a
while he would stop and breathe in the   *81*
wonderful fragrances and get lost in
the splendid colors that surrounded
him.   *80*

Now, (client's name), let that nice
feeling go down the front part of your
body, first down your face, and then   *79*
continuing down your chest, very
pleasant and comfortable feeling, that's
the way. Feeling your chest go up and   *78*
down as you take in refreshing breaths
of air. Letting that pleasant feeling go
all the way down to your stomach.   *77*

Stepping from one aisle to another
he felt enveloped by plants hanging
from above and those down below, a   *76*
profusion of colors and various odors
that soon blended together into one
remarkable humid scent that he soon   *75*
forgot to pay attention to.

Doing very well, (client's name),
slowing down and relaxing your mind   *74*
and your body, and letting that warm
feeling continue now, down those
arms, first that right arm, starting up at   *73*
the shoulder, and going down that arm,
slowly, comfortably, all the way down
that arm to the tips of those fingers.   *72*

In whatever direction the young
man turned, he could see, smell, and
almost feel the growth of these extraor-   *71*
dinary plants. He lost track of time

while he breathed in his surroundings, absorbed in the greenhouse, inwardly *70* amused that his attention could be engaged while time on a clock seemed suspended. *69*

And down that left arm now, (client's name), all the way down your arm. Each part of your body that is touched *68* by this comfortable feeling immediately becomes more and more slowed down and relaxed. Slowing down your *67* mind and your body.

One of the young man's main jobs in the greenhouse was taking little seed- *66* lings from one pot and putting them in a bigger pot. He did this every day at a bench. Little did he know that several *65* months before, someone had accidentally knocked a little seedling off the back of the bench, and there it lay, in *64* the dark, forgotten, apparently lifeless.

And your legs now, starting with your right leg, imagining, just imagin- *63* ing that comfortable feeling going all the way down that right leg, from the hip all the way down past your knee *62* and down to the tips of those toes, just letting it happen, enjoying relaxation and comfort in that leg. *61*

One day the young man found the seedling. He examined it closely and saw the broken pot and dry brown *60* stem on top. The boss was passing by and he casually asked him if he could keep the dry seedling, and the boss *59* said, "Just throw it out. You can have a good one, one that's alive." But the young man persisted and got to keep *58* the little seedling.

And your left leg now, letting that warmth and comfort extend all the way down from your hip down to your knee and beyond, all the way down to the tips of those toes, that's the way.

57

56

At the end of the day the young man examined the little seedling more carefully. He broke away the pieces of the pot and saw that down at the base of the root ball there were little bits of green. The seedling was not dead. In fact, way down there, it was very much alive. All because of its *strong root system*.

55

54

53

All of your body now is totally and comfortably relaxed. Your mind and your body, deeply and comfortably relaxed.

52

He took that little seedling and put it in new soil. He gave it room to grow and water and light of its own. And soon it began to grow. In no time it began to send out new growth above the soil. And it continued to grow, *stronger and stronger*. The little seedling had developed a *strong root system* indeed.

51

50

49

Isn't it nice to know that you can enjoy deep comfort and relaxation, just by imagining, imagining that comfortable feeling slowing down both your mind and your body? You can imagine this any time you like.

48

47

Soon that little seedling developed into a fine tree. And even today it is probably a very nice tree in somebody's yard. After all, that little seedling survived, endured and finally prospered— all because of its *strong root system*.

46

45

Deepening

No additional deepening is usually necessary.

REALERTING

Prior to a quick realerting (e.g., "We're stopping now, so please wake up"), we prefer to suggest amnesia, which can be done in a variety of ways: directly, "You may now forget anything that you may have intended to remember"; metaphorically, "I had a dream last night and when I woke up I could remember only a small part of that dream, or none of it, I cannot recall"; or by offering statements that the client must reflexively answer "no" to, e.g., "It never gets hot in Phoenix," or "*People* magazine never has any pictures in it." With clients in the V.A. we like to say things like "At any V.A. hospital, you never have to wait for an appointment," or "At every V.A., you can never find a cigarette butt outside, or a paper clip inside." Another distraction that fosters amnesia is when, *immediately* after realerting, you question the client about something irrelevant or unrelated, e.g., "Did you see the governor on the news last night?"

Any kind of distraction can cause temporary confusion, and amnesia often follows. Erickson was said to launch into a story about a shaggy dog or, at the end of trance, quickly realert clients and hustle them to the waiting room. In order to be respectful, it is wise to explain to clients that you are doing so-and-so in an effort to help them or to "get in underneath the radar," which many people understand and appreciate.

DEBRIEFING

With clients who are somatic it is important to direct questions to feelings in their bodies. Noticing relaxation, as contrasted with tension or pain, is strongly reinforcing and ratifies trance. If they do not remember the story, frame amnesia as a good hypnotic talent, which, of course, it is. Some concrete clients may feel that they have somehow failed if they cannot remember. We also readily explain the rationale for inducing amnesia: "So it can work in your unconscious mind without interference from your conscious mind."

NOTES FOR PRACTICE

Some may recognize that this greenhouse story was adapted from "The Seedling," a story in Lee Wallas's excellent *Stories for the Third*

Ear (1985). Either story can stand alone, with a more conventional induction, as an ego-strengthening story, or part of therapy. We have found this story and similar ones to be highly potent in "building up" clients, who often voice compelling positive response shortly afterward.

This induction has several distinct advantages. It contains induction, deepening, and therapy. It can also be used several times with the same client, as it is sufficiently "busy." Because people *like it* (they feel better because of it, it stimulates the unconscious, etc.), they do not become bored if you use it on different occasions. In fact, people often report new learnings with subsequent use.

The therapist may experiment with different anchors, such as a fist or a circle with the thumb and forefinger. Use of the anchor in the natural environment should stimulate both relaxation and ego-strengthening. We commonly make tapes for clients to practice at home.

Clients sometimes become lost in the counting and may mix up the numbers, but this doesn't really matter. If they follow instructions to count very slowly, the therapist will finish before they do. If they finish counting early, just have them start again from 100.

PTSD clients prone to dissociation seem to dissociate less with this induction, perhaps because it is sufficiently structured. However, if they do dissociate briefly, gentle redirection to the counting helps them get back on track. If they dissociate for longer periods of time, it may be necessary to suspend the entire process. The structure of this induction also seems to keep intrusive thoughts and similar phenomena contained. In our experience, if PTSD clients are prone to re-experiencing or arousal in trance, the behavior will occur with any induction and even conventional progressive muscle relaxation.

We term this induction "confusional" because of its bilateral process and the opportunity it affords for metaphorical suggestion. Of course, other confusional inductions rely more on word play and overt cognitive overload and confusion.

Some clients who respond favorably to such supportive hypnotherapy are prepared for an exposure-type therapy such as flooding, hypnotic age regression with abreaction and reframing, or eye movement desensitization and reprocessing (EMDR). However, these clients, like many with PTSD, decline any directive treatment for PTSD because they cannot tolerate reopening old wounds.

MYSTIFYING

If a client says, "No, I'm not interested in hypnosis," then we would probably not expend more energy in that direction. However, if the client says, "I want to go into trance *but I just can't*," we have a number of options available. The uninterested client is an example of conscious resistance, while the second client characterizes unconscious resistance.

A two-operator induction may be the quickest route to counter unconscious resistance. However, if you don't have the luxury of a second therapist, this induction may be precisely what you need. Many colleagues have used this induction, and they have told us that it seems to be so bewildering that clients invariably escape into trance. We developed this induction for a young man with Reiter's syndrome, a painful and debilitating form of arthritis. The client badly wanted to go into trance and he said, "Something is holding me back—I don't know what." Since then we have used it with other, less resistant clients. As with all inductions, we tell the person ahead of time what to expect. Then they understand that these strange and seemingly incomprehensible things are being said for their benefit. In other words, we may say, "I'm going to read you something we call 'The Mystifying Induction.'"

A story within a story—or an induction within an induction—is a handy device for bypassing a fixed conscious set. Notice that the suggestion of hypnotic phenomena (e.g., the emphasis on ideosensory feeling) is similar to other inductions, but here overload and confusion are the means of delivery.

We have a hard time remembering this one, so we invariably read it. Before starting, the client is instructed to pick out a spot to look at and to keep looking at that spot while we read the induction. He or she is also told, "You may close your eyes at any time," along with a measure of restraint: "You may go into trance at any time, or simply just listen to the following."

Induction

I want to tell you about a rather strange and bewildering experience one of our therapists had as (s)he went about inducing trance in a person in whom it was rather difficult to distinguish what was happening inside (her) him. Accordingly, the therapist resorted to juxtaposing and mixing up various opposite phenomena in order to induce the desired state. All this might not make sense to you right now, but by the time we're done, you may definitely feel in your own way, or sense in your body, the meaning of what follows.

You know how it is when you're glad you do something, looking back on the experience, maybe appreciating it with the perspective of time or distance. Well, we're glad that we tape recorded the exact words that day, which I will read verbatim to you now.

"Bob"—his name was Bob—"I know and you know and many others know that you and I and most everybody else has a right hand and a left hand, a left foot and a right foot, a right ear and a left, and a conscious mind as well as an unconscious mind.

"With all those things we have many experiences, even way back there, when we learned to count, one, two, three . . . perhaps experiencing a certain feeling or sensation on one side as opposed to the other, or maybe both at the same time. Now, Bob, one time I was working with a man who insisted on being called by his last name, which was Inskeep, a rather uncommon name.

"I said, 'Inskeep, right now I would like you to imagine, just imagine without any conscious effort, a tingling in your left hand for just a moment, and then imagine that tingling in your right hand. That's the way, Inskeep: don't do it, just imagine it. And now we're going to speed it up just a bit, quick now, imagine a tingling in your left earlobe and then the same thing in your right earlobe, and then a numbness, or a tingling, in the left third of your right hand and a tingling, or a numbness, in the right third of your left hand. Autonomy, independence, out there, that's right. I know all this may sound confusing, but just keep on like you're doing, no conscious effort is required at all, and whatever you feel in any of your extremities is just fine, and pay careful attention with your mind.'

"Inskeep was sitting in a chair just like that, Bob, and he told me that as we talked about his hands he was having a difficult time curling up his toes inside his shoes, interesting as that might sound . . . or feel.

"We continued then: 'Inskeep, cold and hot, hot and cold, and the many temperatures in between, eighty degrees, thirty degrees, seventy-five degrees, forty-three degrees, and no one needs a master's degree to feel any of those things. People can develop a light trance or medium trance or a deep trance, whatever their unconscious mind desires, even though sometimes the conscious mind might try to interpose something different. Just imagine, Inskeep, just imagine for a moment a lightness in most of your right hand and a heaviness down there in the bottom part of your left foot. Right hand, left foot, most of up here and bottom part down there, very good, and then a heaviness in a third of your left hand and a lightness in your right foot—not all of your left foot but in just a meaningful part of it. Lightness, heaviness, up here, down there, not all of, just a part of, doing fine, just imagining and knowing that strength means strong mind that can't not possibly not ever resist not drifting off.

"'Inskeep, going inside, a person can pay attention to outside things at the same time, without even trying, independently. Imagine a heavy rubber glove on one hand and a soft warm mitten on the other, either the left or the right, and imagine reaching down and touching a part of your foot that has a numbness, or a tingling, or on the other hand, imagine a heavy woolen sock on one foot, perhaps the left or the right, and reaching that foot up there to touch one of those hands that has developed a particular warmth, or coldness, maybe a tingling warmth, or a numbing coldness in either or maybe both. Someone said to me once that extremities have deep meaning, but I know that not knowing, forgetting, or partially realizing in a light or medium way, out there, is something that also provides something worth noticing, and whatever happens in your body is just fine. But, Inskeep, I personally have no authority to permit your mind to drift, so just concentrate on your body.'"

Bob had been paying close attention and by now had experienced many things in his extremities, but he had also noticed how his breathing had changed almost imperceptibly. He told me later that this experience was not unlike something he remembered when he was very young, filling up a plastic bucket on the beach, and the bucket very quickly filled with sand and overflowed, while the hole in the ground filled with water, and the more he dug, both the bucket and the hole overflowed, and all he learned from the experience was that forever after whenever he met someone named Doug he felt almost overloaded—whatever that means.

Bob also had a teacher in junior high whose last name was Duggin. Mr. Duggin would catch him daydreaming out there in the back row and say to him, "Drift off on your time, Bob, not mine."

"'Inskeep', I continued, 'just imagine my voice is out there along with your extremities, and we'll go on, but a bit faster because now we're nearing the end, and paying close attention now to both out-side and inside might take on an even more curious aspect, or your unconscious mind might just have fun inwardly.

"'Just imagine, Inskeep, the following: a person's left third of his right ear can *now* develop a very distinct feeling, while at the same time the lower part of his left ear can detect the opposite feeling, perhaps alternately, maybe together, always listening, while at the same time he listens inwardly with his third ear, and you know what that is.

"'And while all that is going on with those ears, you can imagine in yourself a left-right, up-down amusement in those hands and feet, while that other person's ears—all three of them—operate independently on their own. Warm-hand-bottom-third or top half with the other cold, and the opposite foot numb or tingling-alternately-left-third-yes-and-rest-of-it-no, or heaviness in one or more parts and one hand that is different from the lightness already present to some degree developing in the other hand or the opposite foot that can't not be taking on a life all its own. Feeling, independence, autonomy, development. . . .'"

Deepening

(Client's name), that's the way. You're doing just fine. Now listen closely as I count down from ten to one and as those numbers descend, down one at a time, you can imagine yourself sinking a bit deeper and deeper into hopefully no more than a light state of trance. Starting to count now: ten . . . nine . . . eight . . . When he was small he blew up a balloon. Was it a green one or a blue one? I for-get. Anyway after blowing it up he stuck his finger into the side of it and wiggled it around, and to this day he wonders if his finger was inside or outside that balloon . . . *you can do it*, (client's name), . . . seven, . . . six . . . The other night I reached for the light switch and it wasn't there . . . and *you can do it*, (client's name), five . . . four . . . three . . . They were selling Mexican blankets alongside the road for only two dollars each . . . and *you can do it*, (client's name), . . . two, and one. . . .

REALERTING

Following the therapy portion, if any, the client is realerted as in the other inductions. As the purpose of a confusional induction is to get the client to experience trance, the induction and deepening alone are usually sufficiently therapeutic for one session.

DEBRIEFING

Post-trance questions should be directed at targets in the induction. "How do you feel in your feet?" "What difference do you notice between your right hand and your left hand?" "You feel woozy in your head? Tell me more about that." Questions such as these, as well as questions directed at time distortion and amnesia, are recommended. All of these things are strong convincers of trance.

NOTES FOR PRACTICE

In the deepening we used the *non sequitur*, a little confusional device that can pay big dividends when parceled out judiciously. Non sequitur is an inference or conclusion that does not follow from the premises, a statement that by itself does not follow or does not fit in the client's conscious set. The result is confusion. People will naturally search for a way out of the confusion, which seems to leave them especially open to suggestion. So, the therapist offers a way out—but in the desired direction. Therefore, *you can do it*, or a similar suggestion is typically advanced, but only after a few seconds, during which time the confusion is allowed to heighten.

Remember that once the client achieves trance you can leave confusional inductions and go to a more conventional one. There are always exceptions, however. The man with Reiter's syndrome *insisted* on this induction forever after. "I really like it," he explained. Over the course of several months we used it as a vehicle for a variety of successful therapeutic applications for pain and anxiety management, ego-strengthening, and increased physical activity.

Once the client successfully experiences trance there is an acceleration of rapport and trust. Cooperation and "the dance" can then begin in earnest, and that is a good time to initiate head nods or finger signalling.

TWO-OPERATOR

Many clients demonstrate increased depth in trance, as well as greater overall responsiveness, with each session of trancework.

Clients begin to feel more comfortable and we can tailor hypno-therapy to their particular needs. They "get better" at hypnosis the more they practice it. Another way to view this is that we are train-ing clients to be good subjects. The clients that Milton Erickson wrote about—those who experienced automatic writing or pseudo-orientation in time, for example—were not uncommon clients. They were ordinary clients with whom Erickson worked very hard, usu-ally for at least eight hours, "training" them in experiencing trance before he attempted certain therapeutic measures that, to many, may seem exotic, or at least difficult to realize.

We employ the two-operator induction with clients who have for-midable unconscious resistance and with whom other inductions have already been attempted. At the Tucson V.A., we do this induc-tion for teaching purposes in our training group, or with chronic, resistant clients who are specifically referred.

We agree ahead of time who will be the "straight man," or the operator who will be offering straightforward suggestions for relax-ation, and who will be the "confuser," or the operator whose confus-ing statements are intended to cause clients to become overloaded so they will escape into trance. We may seed "escape" in pre-trance dis-cussion by casually talking to each other about a movie in which there was an *escape* route or *escape* hatch.

Of course, the client is given the rationale for this induction: "We will both be talking to you at different times, and some of it may seem confusing or not make sense, but this is all done to help you." The client is given permissive instruction regarding eye fixation or closure, and then told to take two deep, cleansing breaths.

Induction

THERAPIST ONE: We are very pleased that you came here today. Now, (client's name), no doubt you *noticed the weather* outside today and you *gave some thought* to what experience you might have here today, wondering whether you might go into a *light* or *medium* trance, recognizing that a deep trance *may not be achievable* at this time.

	truisms
	bind of comparable alternatives
	restraint

THERAPIST TWO: *Don't listen to him.*   *confusion*

THERAPIST ONE: Waiting *out* there   *apposition of opposites*
before coming *in* here, perhaps you
contemplated certain things, and going   *truism*
inside, *to the extent that you can do it*,   *restraint*
may be a very *interesting experience . . .*   *implication*
and whatever kind of experience you
have here today, it is yours and yours
alone to enjoy and appreciate, always
in the driver's seat. . . .   *metaphor*

THERAPIST TWO: *Why do streams run*   *non sequitur/*
day and night in ceaseless flow?   *confusion*

THERAPIST ONE: Doing just fine,
(client's name), *absolutely nothing* at all   *not knowing/not doing*
that a person has to do, or know, or
feel, or think about. . . . *You may be*   *implication*
interested in knowing that some people
who come in here *do not even listen* to   *bind of comparable*
the words, or *tune out* the words,   *alternatives*
totally ignore them, or just *pay atten-*
tion to something else, and even some
just let it go and *have fun* inwardly.

THERAPIST TWO: *He usually tells peo-*
ple, "Please don't listen to the words" . . .   *confusion*
but he doesn't know what he's talking
about.

THERAPIST ONE: *A man* one time   *metaphor*
came in here and sat in that exact chair
and he slowly began to relax, starting
up at his neck and going all down his
body, muscles relaxing, down his arms,
and then his back . . . going deeper and
deeper into a very light and pleasant
state of relaxation. . . .

THERAPIST TWO: *He entered the small silences between the leaves.*

non sequitur/ confusion

THERAPIST ONE: *Another man* started at the bottom, first feeling that pleasant relaxation—or was it a tingling or numbness or some other curious sensation?—in his feet, slowly moving up his legs, just noticing, and eventually appreciating ... comfort and relaxation. ...

metaphor

THERAPIST TWO: *Trance isn't a subjective state anyway.*

confusion

THERAPIST ONE: Still *another person* entertained the idea of *deep trance* versus moderate trance, and another *mild trance* versus the two deeper states, and he eventually decided to make *no conscious decision* at all, and to *just let* himself drift into the depth of trance that was comfortable for him at that time. ...

metaphor

conscious-unconscious double bind

THERAPIST TWO: *You need to watch out for manipulation ... and he may not know what he's talking about ...*

confusion

THERAPIST ONE: Breathing comfortably and relaxed, recognizing how nice and comfortable slowing down can be . . . appreciating those feelings in your body. ...

THERAPIST TWO: *You'll have to drive fast on the way home, so why slow down now?*

confusion

THERAPIST ONE: Going into trance can be especially comfortable, noticing certain feelings in your body . . . and your breathing, noticing—and appreciating—even subtle changes in your breathing, and *how each comfortable breath can take you deeper* and deeper into a light, or even moderate, state of relaxation . . . *and* also noticing how time *might seem to slow down, or speed up*, but time on a clock and time in trance can both become misconstrued, and in the end none of this may matter at all . . . and whether it's losing track of time, or losing the feeling in *that* hand, all these are common experiences in trance. . . .

implication

linking word
time distortion

dissociation

(Therapist One signals for Therapist Two to cease)

THERAPIST ONE: (Client's name), I want you now to just continue as you are, maybe wondering . . . or perhaps your mind is wandering, I don't know, and it *really doesn't matter that you do anything at all*, and I'm going to tell you a little story soon, a story that *may or may not have anything to do with your situation*, and of course, you *may choose to not even listen*, which is just fine. *Some people, coming* in here today like you did *sitting* there and *breathing* in and out like that, and *being aware* of certain feelings in their body, *they* just let themselves drift along while watching a movie, or driving a car, or listening to a story, or anything else, letting their unconscious minds examine and

not knowing/not doing

restraint

metaphor

truisms
metaphor

sort out, in its own way and in its own time, anything that may be important, while *other people* consciously put their minds to the task of letting go, something that certainly requires its own *strength and determination* . . . and in your case it may be too early to tell if your *conscious mind or your unconscious mind* will permit you the comfort and peacefulness of the trance experience, which is really something that *happens all by itself*, like a foot, or a leg falling asleep, or like dozing off when you're tired. . . .

metaphor

reframe

involuntariness

Deepening

THERAPIST ONE: I would like you now to let your experience deepen as I tell you a little story. With stories like this, some people find it interesting to not pay conscious attention to the words while they let their minds drift and dream, or concentrate instead on something else going on outside, or maybe inside. This story, which we call "The Balloons Story," I think it may have been in the late 1950s or thereabouts, a young woman named Maria graduated from a small high school in rural Texas, or it may have been some other state, I'm not sure. In those days, women Maria's age were expected to stay close to home, marry, raise a family; and boys back then were supposed to stay in town, maybe go to work in the filling station, and never stray too far from home. However, Maria was independent and adventurous, as well as very intelligent, and she received a scholarship to study biology at the University of Wisconsin. People back home continued to be surprised by Maria as she went on to medical school and later became a famous researcher, but that really has nothing to do with this story.

As a freshman in Madison, Wisconsin, money was tight and she had to work at different jobs just to make ends meet. She worked whenever she wasn't studying, and among her jobs was selling concessions at University sporting events. She sold hot chocolate, coffee, peanut brittle, and wherever she was assigned, that's where she went, and she always did a very good job. The day of the home-coming football game, the boss said to Maria, "I have a special duty for you today," and he took her down on the field. In the corner of the end zone Maria saw a massive net bulging with hundreds of thousands of small balloons. There were red ones, white ones, green ones, different colors, and all were straining there beneath that towering net.

The boss said, "Maria, your one job is this: When our players run back on the field at the end of the half, you pull this cord and *let all those balloons go*. Just let 'er rip. You understand?" Maria nodded. Certainly this was a very easy job. Just pull that cord. But immediately she began to think to herself, "There must be other ways to *let those balloons go*."

She had never been much of a football fan, so she ignored the game as she looked more closely at all those balloons. She vigorously rubbed her hands together to stay warm, she stamped her feet on the ground, and through the icy vapor of her breath she studied that mountain of balloons. She wondered what it would be like to release just one red balloon, and after opening up sufficient room in the net, she *let it go*. The balloon quickly rose up in the frigid air and soon the swift currents carried it out of the stadium. Maria dashed around to the other side of the net and did the same with a green balloon, opened up the net and just *let it go*. No one paid any attention to Maria, as the Wisconsin Badgers were driving toward the other end zone with less than two minutes until half time.

She giggled as she reached up and let go a white balloon, and then two red ones; then three blue ones over there, and a green one down here. She just *let them go*. She continued in this way, different combinations of colors, two here, five there, up, down, around the other side, delighting in just letting them go. She forgot all about the chilly weather and totally lost track of time, which really doesn't matter because two minutes of clock time in a football game can drag out to ten minutes or more.

At the end of the half the fans roared as the players streamed back on to the field, but Maria heard nothing as she was so engrossed in releasing the balloons. The boss finally got her attention and yelled, "Let 'er rip!" She pulled the cord and all the remaining balloons, thousands and thousands of them, she just *let them go*. . . .

REALERTING

Keeping in mind that our goal is to bypass resistance, we may realert in the following way, which offers a restraining message, praise for a job well done, and a posthypnotic suggestion: "Words being mere words, stories being but many words strung together . . . and sometimes we attach too much meaning to many of these things. At any rate, it's important to recognize the good job you did here today, and we know that the next time you return here, just sitting down there, that can be a signal to you to begin your return once again to the comfort and relaxation of trance."

DEBRIEFING

Responsive clients will show immobility, facial mask, lack of swallowing, and other signs of trance. These convincers of trance need to be ratified along with time distortion and amnesia. Unresponsive clients will not show these behaviors, and these clients may be asked questions about their imaginal or overall subjective experience, e.g., "What was going on inside during this experience?" If they report any absorption—or even curiosity or fascination—at all on this level, we would build the next session around this experience. Some clients may report neither of the above, but will indicate that the two-operator experience was in some way interesting or helpful. This may mean nothing more than an appreciation of our effort to help them achieve trance. If they report that the experience was interesting or helpful, we would repeat the Two-Operator induction next time, perhaps altering it a bit by including longer periods of silence to enhance absorption.

Above all, try not to convey to clients that they have failed. Even if their only "responsive" behavior was sitting there the whole time, emphasize this as something positive that can be built on next time.

NOTES FOR PRACTICE

Over the years we have experimented with this induction in a variety of ways. Both operators speaking at the same time does not appear to be as effective as speaking alternately. We think that speaking simultaneously might be *too* overloading, which may cause the client to escape into resentment rather than trance. With the confuser's role we have tried reading something seemingly nonsensical and confusing, like e.e. cummings' poetry, which produces good results. It is also effective if the confuser alternates a restraining confusional directive ("Don't listen to him") with a non sequitur ("I still wonder why the picture on the wall was crooked"). Both suggestions are confusing and will cause the client to escape in the direction of trance; however, using the alternating non sequitur may soften the relative harshness of the induction, and may also provide imaginal stimulation.

We often use "The Balloons Story" early in therapy, especially with anxious clients. After an induction and deepening we typically set up finger signals for yes, no, and I-don't-know/not ready-to-answer-yet responses. We tell the story, and then ask unconsciously directed questions for clients to answer with finger signals, e.g., "Is this story something that your unconscious mind can put to use? Taking as much time as you need, you may answer with one of your fingers. . . ." In the Two-Operator induction we use "Balloons," or a similar story, as a deepening, because many resistant clients are more easily absorbed in a story than in a standard deepening.

Your goal in this induction is to make trance the most desirable option. All of your efforts are directed at distracting and overloading clients so they escape in the direction of the "straight" operator. Accordingly, you do not want to switch roles during the induction because you want clients to become wedded to the "straight" operator. In doing this with one operator, you would need to switch chairs and consequently alter your voice each time. This is unwieldy, as is having the confuser's part on a tape recorder, although some of our colleagues have done this successfully. The availability of two operators is a luxury in most settings; however, arranging this is well worth the effort, as many clients respond very well to two voices, even with standard inductions.

At this point some of you may be thinking, "I don't want to go to all that trouble to put someone in trance." In that case, try the Mystifying induction first. It often works as well as this one. Remember, many resistant clients will respond well to the effort you expend in an induction such as this one, and at that point you have successfully cut throught their resistance. Next session, you can return to one of your standard inductions.

LEFT-RIGHT

Citrenbaum, King, and Cohen (1985) describe how one day the three authors got lost on the way to conduct a workshop. They stopped to ask directions at a gas station and were told, "It's two lefts and three rights." The trio became hopelessly confused and lost their way, but the experience taught them something about letting go. We have adapted this anecdote into a confusional induction and then employ a story we call "Simple Rooms" as a vehicle for deepening.

As with the other confusional inductions, we resort to these when other inductions have not achieved trance. It reminds us of the treatment of tuberculosis (TB) in the first half of this century. The V.A. Medical Center in Tucson, built as a TB hospital in 1920, is an attractive, tiled-roof complex modeled after a nearby Spanish mission from the 1600s. Its open-air rooftops are walkways now, but back then patients spent a good part of the day there, as sitting in the sun was one of the primary treatments for TB in those days. Prior to the advent of effective pharmaceutical agents, TB patients would move to Arizona, gasp and cough up on the roof. If sunshine, rest, and good nutrition did not work, surgeons removed infected ribs and portions of lungs. Some patients got better, and some did not. Treatment options were few, and when treatment failed, all doctors could really do was *more of the same*. Pharmaceuticals were eventually available to treat the disease, and if a patient was refractory to one drug, there were others to try, including experimental agents.

During the same era, psychotherapy and hypnosis consisted in large part of long-term psychoanalytic therapy and highly directive techniques in hypnosis. Treatment options were few, and if something did not work, psychotherapists invariably turned to *more of the same*. Prodigious thinkers like B.F. Skinner and Milton Erickson may not have had as great an impact as life-saving drugs, but their influence has been considerable. We now have many more approaches, such as confusional inductions, to treat clients who are refractory to first-line approaches.

In the deepening we employ a story called "Simple Rooms," which is adapted from a teaching tale that Erickson called "Going from Room to Room" (Rosen, 1982). The meta-message in the story is that *there are many ways to get from here to there*. Throughout this story we ask clients to let themselves sink deeper into trance, but only for a short time. They are then asked to lighten their experience and turn their attention to the story once again.

With these inductions it is always important to explain the rationale for your "crazy-sounding" methods, so that clients don't perceive you as disrespectful. Clients who may not understand concepts such as unconscious resistance will understand "trying something interesting and unusual in order to help them go into trance."

Induction

One afternoon a woman set out looking for her friend's house. She was feeling rather tired and sleepy, but perked up halfway there when she realized she'd forgotten the directions. She decided to check for the directions anyway, and holding the wheel with her left hand she placed the Diet Rite Cola on the floor with her right hand, and reached across to her left coat pocket for the directions, which weren't there. They weren't in her other pockets either, which she checked thoroughly with both hands alternately as she steadied the wheel with one knee and then the other. Then she remembered that her friend had said, "It's two rights and one left."

She took a right and was left with one right and one left. She took a left and was still left with one left and two rights. She tried two rights and was left with the one left, and after trying just one left alone, was left with two rights, and *still* she had not found her friend's house, which was starting to get just a bit confusing.

She decided to try even harder, which was hard as she fought off fatigue and the traffic, and the first thing she did was reverse the right-left order, which she definitely thought was the right thing to do just then. Leaving from the corner she took a hard left, leaving two rights left, and still she was not there. A right and a left, and continuing with one more right left her not there yet either, and finally, in utter bewilderment and near exasperation, she pulled off the road, sat back behind the wheel, took one deep breath, and said, "Oh, well, I might as well just *let it go*."

Deepening

(Client's name), we now enter the deepening portion of trancework today. What I'm going to do is tell you a little story called "Simple

Rooms." I'd like you to listen to this story, but it's not necessary to listen too closely to it, as sometimes we tend to attach unnecessary meaning to certain stories, and maybe to our experiences in general. Throughout the story, I'm going to be giving you some special instructions to allow your experience to deepen. It is all very easy, and you may find it rather interesting. When you are ready to proceed, let me know by nodding your head . . . good.

One day a person—let's call him Sanchez—he came inside, from out in the cold, and said he was having difficulty getting *from here to there*. So, I asked him, "Sanchez, in your house over on the northeast side of town, how would you get from *one room to another*?" He then recounted all the possible ways he could think of for getting from *one room to another*. He said he could walk in, crawl in on his knees, or he could somersault through the doorway.

(Client's name), okay, I'd like you now to take one deep breath and let yourself sink deeper into trance . . . that's the way . . . enjoying deeper comfort and relaxation . . . and *now* leave that comfort and relaxation for another time and return to listening to the story . . . good.

And he said he could also go in backwards, or scoot in on his belly, or even on his back. He could enter slowly, or quickly, or with his back—or his chest—up against one door jamb or the other. Maybe he could even put a ladder in the doorway.

(Client's name), doing just fine . . . and now I'd like you to take one deep breath and let yourself sink deeper and deeper into trance . . . enjoying deeper comfort and relaxation, perhaps deeper than ever before, I don't know . . . and *now* leave that comfort and relaxation for another time and return to listening to the story. . . .

And Sanchez also said he could *go from one room to another* with big steps, medium steps, or small steps, and even on tiptoes. He could go around the house and climb in the back window. He even mentioned various other things that I can't remember. Finally, after several minutes of some real hard brainstorming of how to *go from one room to another*, he had exhausted all the possible ways *to get from here to there*.

(Client's name), okay, now I'd like you one more time to take that deep breath and let yourself sink deeper into trance . . . enjoying deeper comfort and relaxation . . . very good . . . and *now* leave that comfort and relaxation for another time and return to listening to that story . . . good.

Upon further reflection, and with some discussion, it came to light that there were actually many other ways *to get from one room to another*. He could go in on the hour, on the half-hour, or at some other time on the clock. He could go in after drinking one quarter glass of diet soda, or a half glass of whole milk; he could go in while listening to something on the radio, or he could *go from one room to another* thinking of something important one time, and leaving his mind blank another time.

He could even walk around the block three times, go to the airport and fly to London and back, and *then* enter that other room. Together we came up with many, many possibilities and I wasn't able to write them all down. One thing that I learned in that experience, as did Sanchez, was that *there are an infinite number of ways to get from one room to another.*

REALERTING

We like to realert rapidly with something like, "I would like you to wake up now, *eyes open*, very good."

DEBRIEFING

Some clients will not remember the deepening story, but they will recall the unpleasantness of having the deepening periods interrupted. General open-ended questions are in order, e.g., "How do you feel?" "What are you thinking?" "Do you remember everything?"

NOTES FOR PRACTICE

A sudden realerting, which may produce amnesia, is recommended to promote unconscious processing, as we discussed earlier. Some clients may remember everything. In such cases, reinforce them for what they *did* accomplish, e.g., eye closure, paying close attention, sitting still, etc. Many times clients who did not experience amnesia wish to discuss the meaning of the story. We never discuss this with clients, preferring instead to not reinforce conscious process. We usually tell clients something like, "Let the back part of your mind work on this for awhile." Clients soon become accustomed to indirection and not discussing metaphors. Clients who do not experience an appreciable depth in trance may return with a new learning or new behavior, and many may be sufficiently prepared for a more conventional induction.

In the deepening we ask for a head nod in order to proceed. Most clients will nod their head. However, clients occasionally may not nod or give a discernible nod. If this happens, say something like, "You're doing fine, recognizing how relaxation can come very comfortably at its own pace, and as we continue, you may experience some very curious things. . . ." Commitment is very important, but not so important that it diverts you from your task. Lingering too long waiting for a head nod, or asking for a verbal report or finger signal instead, may signal power struggle to the client, and it is more important to proceed.

In the deepening we intentionally withhold something pleasant from the client. In building responsiveness in hypnosis, or in psychotherapy in general, people may appreciate something more if it does not come too easily.

5

Directive Inductions

ARM CATALEPSY

Sometimes called Catalepsy, this induction is one that clinicians will often see in live demonstrations. Several years ago I (GG) was in the audience at a large conference, and D. Corydon Hammond used this induction with a male subject who had suffered sexual abuse. Dr. Hammond readily induced trance in the client, then progressed to age regression, abreaction, and reframing, an effective hypnotic technique for treating trauma.

This induction is very fast, providing quick trance ratification. It should not be used with clients who fear losing control. For some clients, it is very disconcerting to see their arm lowering or raising involuntarily, in response to the wish of their unconscious mind. You begin by asking which is the preferred or dominant hand. You may then seed the response by telling the client, "Hold that right arm straight out in front of you. How does that feel? Good, you may now rest that hand again on your lap."

In early sessions with new clients, it is important to mention the concept of the unconscious mind ahead of time. With some clients a more useful term may be "subconscious mind," "back part of the mind," or even "your imagination."

Induction

(Gently taking the client's hand and holding it from underneath) I'm going to take your hand and hold it right out here like this . . . and I'd like you to *pick out a spot* to look at on the back of *that hand*, and when you've selected a spot, let me know by nodding your head . . . good.

eye fixation

dissociative language

(Slowly letting go of the hand) I'm going to let *that hand* float right out there like that, that's the way. Now maybe *that hand* feels heavy, maybe light, I don't know, and *it has little quivering movements* and we don't know yet if the *lightness* in that hand will cause it to *float up* to your face or if the *heaviness* in that hand will allow it to *sink down* to the comfort of your lap, and it really doesn't matter, as there's absolutely *nothing at all that you have to consciously do, or know, or think about or change* . . . little *shaking movements, moving downward* a bit at a time.

pacing

permissive suggestion

not knowing/not doing

pacing

Doing this exercise here today, and *perhaps noticing your breathing*, and becoming more and more *absorbed in that spot* on the back of your hand as it seems to be moving ever so slowly downward, I want you to *not let that hand sink down to the comfort of your lap until your unconscious mind is ready for you to go* into a nice, deep

truisms

contingent suggestion

trance, that's the way . . . little *sinking movements* ever downward.

(Client's hand touches lap) Very good. (If client has not already closed his eyes) Now just let those *eyes gently close and sit back* in that chair.

pacing

suggestion

Deepening

(Client's name), I'd like to take a few moments to let your experience deepen . . . (waiting 30 seconds or so) and now I'd like you to take two more deep, refreshing breaths to let yourself sink even deeper and deeper into a very profound and restful state of relaxation . . . and when you are sufficiently deep, your unconscious mind will know because your right index finger will twitch and develop a lightness all its own and move up into the air. Allow your unconscious mind as much time as it needs. . . .

REALERTING

Following therapy, the client is realerted by counting from one to five.

DEBRIEFING

Time distortion should be targeted following this induction, as clients invariably believe that much more time has passed than has actually passed in clock time, e.g., "Without looking at the clock on the wall, please take a guess at what time you think it is right now." Querying regarding ideosensory feelings often yields a feeling of heaviness in the cataleptic arm.

NOTES FOR PRACTICE

The vast majority of clients' hands will sink down rather than float up; however, the therapist needs to be prepared to pace the response in case it goes up. In that case, the unconsciously-directed suggestion would be, ". . . until that hand touches your face."

I (GG) had a client once whose hand sank down to one inch above her lap, and there it floated for some 20 minutes as I was starting to run out of things to say. Finally, she opened her eyes and remarked,

"Am I fighting you?" This was an important lesson for me, in that it demonstrated the potency of her unconscious resistance. When that happened later with subsequent clients, I simply told them to "put your unconscious mind on hold for now and just rest that hand back on your lap." In recent years I've only used this induction for demonstration purposes in our training group or with clients who express a strong need to experience involuntariness.

You will notice that, in the deepening, a finger signal was requested in response to an *unconscious* suggestion. If the client had not responded positively to the unconscious suggestion during the induction, then I would have asked for a response that was implicitly *conscious*, a head nod or a finger signal: "When you are sufficiently deep, you may let me know by raising your right index finger." These responses usually involve a deliberate raising of the finger a few inches in the air, while a true unconscious response is usually a mere twitch or quiver. Whenever any kind of finger signalling will be done during the session, ask the client to place her hands on her lap when you start. Otherwise, finger movements will be difficult to see.

This induction is contraindicated in people with neck or back pain—another reason to ask them to extend their arm and ask them how that feels before you begin.

STIFF ARM

Highly directive inductions are strong, fast ratifiers of trance. This induction, which is also referred to as Limb Rigidity or Arm Rigidity, is used by Crasilneck (1982) in the treatment of erectile dysfunction, or as part of a constellation of similar techniques (e.g., glove anesthesia, hand levitation) in the treatment of warts (Crasilneck & Hall, 1985). Clients who experience involuntariness (e.g., a stiff arm that cannot be bent) may be convinced of the power of hypnosis and their own mind to stimulate erections or remove warts (Hammond, 1990). In this book we have underscored the importance of ratifying trance as a convincer. Nevertheless, another significant byproduct of trance ratification is that it counters discouragement and provides hope by demonstrating that change is possible (Hammond, 1990).

With this induction, it helps to hold the client's arm once it becomes stiff. Accordingly, we like to first ask for permission to do so. Also, we ask the client to rehearse the behavior ahead of time: "Do this for me, please. Hold out your right (preferred) arm like this and make a fist . . . good, how does that feel? Okay, you may relax your arm again. . . ." In case you have overlooked cervical pain, peripheral neuropathy, or a similar condition, this brief rehearsal both checks for pain and seeds the response.

The brief induction is followed by a longer deepening story that we use in the initial stages of treating psychogenic erectile dysfunction or impotence. Letters of the alphabet and numbers are employed as part of various indirect suggestions for mastery, rigidity, and strength. Because catalepsy characterizes impotence, *movement* is suggested in these letters and numbers, which include six and nine, two numbers with a sexual connotation, and three, which connotes "third leg," or penis.

Induction

(Therapist sits a few feet in front of client.)

Stretch out that right arm for me again, that's the way, and make a strong fist, very good.

I'm going to touch your arm now, and as I do so I want you to make that arm tight, strong, like a bar of steel, good. . . .

therapist touches arm

Make that arm stronger and stronger, so that it cannot be bent, like a bar of steel, like a piece of wood soaked in water for several days, and now it's hard, strong, unbendable, and I'm going to try and bend it now and I can't because it's so very hard and strong, like a bar of steel. Never before have you made something so strong, so hard. This shows the power of your unconscious mind, and you can put this power to good use beginning now . . . very good.

therapist tries to bend arm

Now, (client's name,) I want you to
slowly relax that arm, and as it returns
to your lap you can sit back, close your
eyes, and let yourself drift off into a
very pleasant and satisfying trance, as I
continue to talk to you . . . and I'm
going to tell you a little tale called "The
Southeast Extension Story. . . ."

Deepening

State of being, state of mind, relaxing in both mind and body. Just
letting go, nothing to do or know, just relaxing into the sound of my
voice. Peaceful and calm, that's the way. . . .

Letting your mind drift and dream, you can think back to some
hard tasks you've mastered in the past . . . perhaps first learning to
write the letters of the alphabet, no doubt a *hard* thing to do, and at
first someone took your hand and helped point the way, and as you
gradually did it yourself perhaps your whole body went into forming
those letters, and maybe you even stuck out the tip of that tongue as
you concentrated on doing it just right. As it became easier for you,
soon you used just your hand, then gradually, you were able to write
easily with just the thumb and first finger or two of your writing
hand. And with practice, your aim, between the lines or wherever
you wrote, was good, and the whole thing became easy, smooth,
automatic, and you didn't have to stop and think anymore what side
the stick was on for the letter B or D. *Did* the stick go up or down for
a P? And how many legs *does* an M have? Is a three just an M on its
side, or is a six an upside down nine, or the other way around? One
time a man made both letters and numbers with wooden match
sticks because they stayed in position longer than paper matches.
Odd things that people do. I think it was that same man who said
that Chinese arithmetic was the hardest thing he had ever mastered.

It can be so very pleasant and comfortable to relax, relaxing your
mind and body. When you came in here you perked up your mind,
paying close attention to everything, and then you let your mind
relax. And your body, too, sometimes it's alert and aroused, and other
times those muscles just relax, noticing the contrast not unlike
asleep and awake, or tense and relaxed, or day and night. Isn't it nice

that while your muscles relax your *bones can remain rigid and strong*, or else you'd fall over, *just like everybody else.*

Strong skyscrapers with those steel poles are certainly rigid, but even they have some flexibility to maintain their structure if the earth begins to quake. People who build *strong buildings* should be proud of their work, and no doubt you can think back on things in the past, maybe recently, maybe long ago, when you were successful accomplishing something, maybe big, maybe small, and there's nothing like feeling good, feeling proud of what you've done.

Just thinking for a moment about sports. In football they used to play both offense and defense for four quarters, and in baseball a pitcher would go for nine innings, but in recent years it's gotten pretty specialized and people play their position for a shorter length of time, and maybe they play *even harder* as a result. I know in basketball sometimes a player will go the whole 40 minutes without a break, but more often players get a nice rest, which they appreciate, and as a result they come back *harder and stronger* once they're back in the game.

REALERTING

Realerting in the following way is designed to promote both amnesia and bodily dissociation or numbness: "(Client's name), we know that *People* magazine has no pictures in it, and Phoenix and Minneapolis have exactly the same climate, and in a moment I'm going to have you reawaken in a very special way as I count from one to five. You can wake up as a mind, but not as a body, and I'm beginning to count now . . . one . . . two . . ."

DEBRIEFING

By immediately directing questions at ideosensory phenomena, you reinforce the "but not as a body," which also serves as a conscious distraction, thus reinforcing the suggestions for amnesia.

NOTES FOR PRACTICE

The inclusion of an embedded-meaning deepening after a highly directive induction should not imply that we are tightly wedded to the indirect. On the contrary, we have found that the two polar approaches complement each other nicely. Highly suggestible clients—those who rapidly develop arm rigidity, sit back, and go deeply into trance—will respond well to both the dissociative double bind realerting and the amnesia-facilitating questions that demand a *no* response. These clients will not only have no memory of the deepening, but may also require extra time to let their bodies fully reawaken before you end the session. It is important to make sure the client is realerted before leaving the session, particularly after using the suggestion of not waking the body. Otherwise problems may arise from decreased reaction time or delayed cognitions.

Very rarely we will encounter a client who does not come out of trance. Helen Watkins (1986) advises repeating calm, firm dehypnotizing suggestions until the client realerts, and then inquiring about feelings and experiences. Such dissociation may be a naturally occurring phenomenon, in which case continued hypnosis may be contraindicated unless the practitioner has expertise with such problems (Dolan, 1991; Kluft, 1993). A fascinating and compelling hypnotherapeutic approach to this and other problems is ego-state therapy. John and Helen Watkins, who pioneered this approach, have articulated it in *Ego States: Theory and Therapy* (1997; see also Phillips & Frederick, 1995).

COIN DROP

This technique, described in the American Society of Clinical Hypnosis manual of inductions (Hammond, 1988), is attributed to Alexander Levitan, M.D. It is a rapid induction that is useful for clients who need validation or feedback that they are entering trance, as well as for clinicians who are first learning how to do inductions. We introduce it early in training as a fast, simple induction. The therapist is required to pay close attention to both pacing and leading. For example, if the client drops the coin before the end of the induction, you must be prepared to pace the response and move on to the next step.

The manner in which the coin is obtained may embellish the process. You ask the client or someone else in the training group: "Does someone have a coin? Any coin will do." The client is then instructed to hold the coin gently between the thumb and forefinger with the wrist flexed downward. The arm is at a right angle to the body. We adapted the following induction from Dr. Levitan's original, and colleague Chris Young provided the deepening.

Induction

I would like you to *focus your attention* on your thumbnail, that's the way. *And* as you are doing so, you can notice the coin *supported by your thumb and fore-finger*, and perhaps you feel your fingers *tingling* around it, or else you may feel *some other interesting or curious sensation* developing out there.

    Now, (client's name), before too long that coin *will grow heavier and heavier*, and at the same time you may feel your eyelids growing heavy *as you continue to gaze at that spot*.

    It may feel very good to *close those eyes whenever you wish*, or else you *may continue to look at that spot*, which can be a very absorbing thing all in itself. *And* as you continue to become more and more relaxed, you can notice how your breathing has begun to change, maybe *speeding up* or *slowing down*, and you can know that *as soon as* you are ready to become even more relaxed, that coin will drop, *all by itself without any conscious effort on your part.*

    And the sound of the coin hitting the floor will tell me and tell you that you have entered a pleasant state of comfort and relaxation. *That's the way*, just letting it happen *all by itself*, taking as much time as you need. . . .

    (As the coin drops) *Very good, doing just fine*. And no doubt your *arm is also feeling heavy*, and it can *slowly move over* to the comfort of your lap, *and as it does so*, you can just *sit back, take one more deep comfortable breath, and let*

eye fixation
linking word

truism

suggestion covering all possibilities

suggestion

pacing

permissive suggestion

linking word

apposition of opposites

contingent suggestion

involuntariness

pacing
involuntariness

pacing

leading

yourself sink even deeper and deeper   *pacing*
into a very satisfying state of trance.
Nothing at all that you need to do or   *not knowing/not doing*
know or think about except experience
this pleasantness, comfort, and relaxation.

Deepening

Now I'd like you imagine, (client's name), that you are in a department store in a city, any city you like. When you can imagine
that, taking as much time as you need, let me know by nodding your
head . . . good. . . . Now this department store happens to have ten
floors, and in a moment I'm going to ask you to descend, in your
mind, down one floor at a time, and with each passing floor, you will
feel even more deeply and comfortably relaxed. I don't know if in
that elevator you are alone or if other people are with you. It's one of
those old fashioned elevators where the elevator operator pulls back
the door at each stop and announces what goods and services can be
found on that floor.

He opens the door at the tenth floor and calls out, "Hair salon,
portrait studios, and a fine view of the city." He closes the door and
announces, "Down we go!"

Soon he calls out, "Ninth floor—vacuums, sewing machines, dish-
washers, and water heaters. Nobody getting out? Okay, down we go!

"Eighth floor—microwaves, refrigerators, freezers, ovens, ranges,
cooktops, and air conditioners. It's cold on the eighth floor. Down we
go!

"Seventh floor—sporting goods, hearing aids, and something else
that I can't recall. Nobody getting out? Then down we go!"

At the sixth floor he adjusts his tie and says softly, "The sixth floor
has housewares, draperies, curtain rods, carpets, and floorcovering.
Down we go!

"Fifth floor—men's shoes, men's wear, boy's wear, outerwear,
innerwear. We're halfway down now.

"Fourth floor has girl's wear, women's wear, takes up the entire
floor. Nobody getting out? Okay, down we go!

"I like this next floor best. Third floor—TVs, stereos, CDs, tapes,
computers, sundry electronics. We'll be down at the bottom soon.
Nobody getting off? Then down we go!

"Second floor—bed and bath, optical, jewelry, fragrances, all kinds of fragrances. I can smell them before we even get there. Down we go!

"First floor—hardware and automotive. We're down as far as you can go on this elevator. But if you want to continue to go down, there are some stairs off to the right. On those stairs you can go down even more."

REALERTING

Following therapy, counting up serves as a useful complement to the deepening. "As I count from one up to five you can feel yourself becoming alert and refreshed, and before I reach five you can open your eyes."

DEBRIEFING

As in the other inductions, it is essential to ratify the trance experience by asking about ideosensory feeling, time distortion, and amnesia. Assessing client response to the directiveness and structure of this induction and deepening is most important. If clients report that they found these elements too gimmicky or too difficult to imagine, consider using a more permissive induction and deepening in subsequent sessions. On the other hand, some clients report total immersion in, and utter fascination with, these techniques, in which case they can be repeated.

NOTES FOR PRACTICE

It is important to remember that this is not just hypnosis, but hypno-*therapy*. You want to find out *what works for the client*. If she responds to the Coin Drop induction along with a permissive period of silence as the deepening, then you have your vehicle, or route, to the objective, which is the therapeutic application. However, if the client likes the Coin Drop, but you want to try something different, we suggest you have the client sit back, close her eyes, and simply *imagine* dropping the coin. This should work equally as well.

HAND LEVITATION

This induction, often demonstrated in workshops, has a special utility as both a training exercise and as a potent convincer of trance for those clients who require an undeniable ratifier. Watching their hand rise strongly reinforces the involuntariness of the experience for clients. In terms of difficulty, we see the Stiff Arm induction as easier to conduct with, perhaps, similar utility. For those of you who are learning new inductions, we encourage finding one or two directive inductions that you are comfortable with, as the comfort and confidence that you convey to your clients will help you inestimably in providing good hypnotherapy.

We precede this induction with a portion of a story that Dr. Mirto Stone used with weight reduction clients when she was an intern in Tucson. The client's attention is absorbed in drinking a cup of tea while the therapist embeds *light* and *slow*, strongly seeding behaviors that are part of Hand Levitation.

The client is asked, for example, "Is it okay if we induce trance today by letting your hand lift up into the air? I think you'll find it very interesting." They are then asked to sit back, place their hands on their lap, close their eyes if they wish, and listen to a story before the induction begins.

Induction

This may be the first time you ever heard a story about a professional tea taster, yes, a tea taster. I'd like you now to just imagine, to just picture in your mind such a person, that tea taster, *raising* a cup of tea, spending a little time, *slowly* looking at the reflections of *light* and color . . . clarity . . . of the tea. That's the way, just imagining, or wondering, can be a very pleasant experience. Breathing in, and breathing out, more and more relaxed and comfortable.

That tea taster *slowly* . . . very *slowly raises* the cup again and spends a few moments noticing . . . appreciating . . . and enjoying the delicate aroma of the tea, and at the same time, you may begin to notice an even deeper de*light*ful state of trance, maybe *lighter* in a deep way or deeper in a *light* way, or something entirely different, I don't know, and it really doesn't matter at all because there's nothing a person needs to think about, or do, or know, or anything else, as you notice and appreciate just how pleasantly relaxed you can become.

Certainly the tea taster derives the utmost de*light* from a small quantity of tea . . . *slowly* . . . breathing in the aroma, just a little sip, which is much different from the person who gulps down the whole cup. *Slowly* taking just a little sip at a time and focusing on the subtle flavors . . . and colors, and noticing the feeling of the tea in your mouth . . . each second is stretched out . . . *slowly* . . . de*light*-fully . . . which for some people could be an en*light*ening experience as well as something very enjoyable and pleasurable.

(Client's name), I'd like you to gently and lightly cup that right (or left, if that is preferred) hand on your lap, just raising up those fingers, and that thumb, so that they are ever so lightly touching your leg . . . and at the same time (if their eyes are open) just focus your attention, with your eyes, on the back of that hand, or (if their eyes remain closed) you can just continue deep relaxation in your body as that hand develops a special lightness all its own . . . that's the way.

You can feel the fabric of your pants/dress beneath those fingers, and that thumb, and perhaps you can begin to detect a warmth or a tingling more in one finger than another, and you can begin to notice very slight, almost imperceptible movements out there, in that hand, and at the same time you can begin to imagine, just imagine, that your hand is becoming very, very light . . . almost light as a feather . . . and as one finger moves first, then the other fingers, and the rest of your hand will follow as it slowly moves up . . . almost as if a balloon up at the ceiling is lifting up that hand, slowly . . . and when that hand touches your forehcad, this will be a sign to you that you can go ever more deeply into a pleasant state of trance . . . that's the way. . . .

(When the hand has touched the forehead—or when it rises as far as it is going to go) . . . very good, and now just let that hand relax again on your lap.

Deepening

In a moment, (client's name), I'm going to count down from ten to one, and each time I say a number out loud, I'd like you to say to yourself, "deeper and deeper." I will begin to count now . . .

REALERTING

Realert the client by counting up from one to five.

DEBRIEFING

Clients are often quite astonished that their hand lifted seemingly all on its own. This should be ratified along with ideosensory feelings, time distortion, and amnesia, if any.

NOTES FOR PRACTICE

Some therapists will very lightly assist the hand in lifting if the hand does not lift following initial suggestions to do so. If you do this, say, "I'm going to reach over now and very gently touch your wrist. . . ." Rendering such assistance usually does not detract from the sense of wonderment experienced when they see their hand levitate seemingly all by itself. In subsequent sessions, clients will usually respond to a conversational or embedded-meaning induction. The self-suggestion in the deepening is also useful with other inductions.

You can tailor this self-suggestion to the particular needs of the client. For clients who desire only a light trance, it may be "deeper and deeper into a light state of trance." For clients who want increased motivation or self-efficacy, you may try, "I can do it" or "I can be strong."

ICE BATH

We have saved one of the most interesting directive inductions for last. Did you ever think of using a bucket of ice water to induce trance? Well, we incorporated it into an induction, not because the ice bath itself induces trance, but because it so strongly *convinces* the client of trance.

Cold pressor pain (immersing a hand in ice cold water) has been used for many years in experimental hypnosis to study such phenomena as hypnotic susceptibility and hypnotic versus waking analgesia (Stam & Spanos, 1980), and the effect of hypnotic analgesia and relaxation on multiple dimensions of pain (Dahlgren, Jurtz, Strube, & Malone, 1995). We do not intend to be scientific here, only to demonstrate the utility of this technique as a hypnotic induction.

We use the Ice Bath induction judiciously and only with clients who express a strong need for proof that they experienced trance. Experiencing time distortion or amnesia is insufficient evidence for these clients. Success with other directive inductions may also be insufficient. They may say, "Show me some proof" or "I need to be convinced that I went under." If the Ice Bath induction does not give them what they are looking for, then we have no stronger convincers. We do not recommend more noxious or invasive stimuli.

You will need a stopwatch or wristwatch, a towel, and a small bucket that is deep enough for clients to immerse their hand up to the middle of the forearm. The bucket is filled with ice and water and placed at a comfortable level next to the client, and the towel is kept on the person's lap. The client understands and agrees with the rationale, and you explain that he/she will first immerse a hand without trance, and then a second time with the benefit of hypnotic induction.

Induction

Ask the client to immerse her hand in the bucket and keep it in as long as she can tolerate it. As the hand is immersed you begin keeping time. After 15 seconds or so, ask the client for a verbal report of pain on a 1–10 scale. When the hand is removed from the bucket, write down the elapsed minutes and seconds and ask again for a scaled subjective level.

The hand is dried and then you induce trance, preferably with a conversational or embedded-meaning induction such as those found in earlier chapters. Draw the induction out, and include a long deepening or story. You may experiment by including images of warmth (a nice summer day at the beach) or various suggestions for analgesia in the immersed hand.

Analgesia may be induced using direct suggestions, "Imagine that hand wearing a warm, heavy, waterproof glove . . . and notice how that glove then reduces the sensations your skin experiences," or by indirect suggestion of numbness such as "and everyone knows what it feels like when a hand falls asleep or when a dentist gives novocaine." Suggesting sensory substitution such as itching or tingling instead of coldness (Barber, 1996), or sensory displacement, e.g., "and some or all of that coldness in your left hand can be shared by your right foot" can also increase the analgesic phenomenon. Finally, either direct or indirect suggestions may be used to increase dissociation. For example, suggesting that the hand is detached from the arm, or that the client is watching the immersed hand from an outside perspective, or imagining the immersed hand as someone else's hand, can all induce dissociation.

When the client appears to be sufficiently deep, ask her to immerse her hand in the bucket again and to keep it in "as long as you can tolerate it." You begin keeping time again and stop as soon as their hand is removed from the bucket. Ask for a verbal report on a 1–10 scale at intervals.

REALERTING

Following this induction, we may say, "You may dry off that hand now and return to your alert state."

DEBRIEFING

Most clients will be able to keep their hand immersed at least two to three times as long with the second immersion. Also, their subjective level of pain will be considerably less. Emphasize to them the differential in time between the two immersions. We like to ask the obvious question at this juncture: "Why do you think there is a difference between the two immersions?" Many clients will respond with utter amazement at their response. Offer praise for a job well done.

NOTES FOR PRACTICE

Clients who have responded favorably are now sufficiently prepared for a more conventional induction in the future. We have never had someone ask for the Ice Bath induction a second time. If clients show no obvious differential (at least 30 seconds or more), emphasize the good job they did anyway. We simply tell these clients that we have nothing else to offer as a strong convincer. We may add, "If strong evidence of trance continues to be important to you, maybe this means your unconscious mind is conveying to you that hypnosis is not something that can help you at this time. Clearly this is something that should be respected. However, you may wish to continue to use hypnosis anyway, setting aside this challenge from your unconscious for a session or two, as sometimes people can make progress on X (presenting problem) while their unconscious mind deliberates possible changes in its position. Or else you may wish to use conventional psychotherapy, or just do nothing for a while to see what happens."

Permissively placing their choice in such a frame often frees clients up to resume hypnosis. If this is what they choose, we can presume that unconscious resistance has already been eroded. Should this induction be used with pain clients? Some of our colleagues say no, as these clients already know how to experience pain. We believe the ice bath induction has utility for any client who needs a strong convincer. If pain clients or any other clients do not have their experience sufficiently ratified, hypnosis may not be effective.

6

Inductions for Children

HYPNOTHERAPY WITH CHILDREN

One of the most poignant accounts we have read is Crasilneck and Hall's (1985) consultation in the case of a four-year-old boy with terminal cancer. The frightened boy refused to eat, and medication and other supportive measures proved futile. The child's hysterical screams were unbearable to both parents and hospital staff, who felt completely helpless. Crasilneck, a seasoned psychologist known for his success with highly directive techniques, engaged his young patient and quickly induced a deep trance by absorbing the boy's attention in the flame of a cigarette lighter. The boy responded favorably to suggestions for relaxation, pain control, and improved sleep and nutrition. An auspicious calm descended on all concerned. Then the boy died, peacefully.

There is a substantial body of literature on the use of hypnosis with childhood medical and other problems. These applications include hematology oncology problems (Jacobs, Pelier, & Larkin,

1998), wart regression (Felt et al., 1998), deafness (Kohen, Mann-Rinehard, Schmitz, & Wills, 1998), and dental phobia (Bird, 1997), to name but a few. The literature is also replete with case reports and studies citing the use of hypnosis for nail biting, thumb sucking, enuresis, situational and phobic disorders, and various other presenting issues (Zahourek, 1985).

Yapko (1990) notes that some practitioners may doubt the hypnotic responsiveness of children because of their own inflexible expectations of how people must behave in trance. A restless or fidgety child, for example, may be very much in trance. Our task is to adapt therapy to children and encourage them to make use of what they do naturally. Psychotherapy with a 14-year-old may consist entirely of talking, just as hypnotherapy with the same adolescent may involve an induction similar to those used with adults. However, "psychotherapy" with a four-year-old will almost always consist of play therapy or a similar modality, and a hypnotherapeutic induction with the same child will likely employ bouncing a ball, storytelling, or similar activity that is natural and age-appropriate. In my (SB) practice, I continue to be fascinated by the number of trance states that children naturally go into and come out of during the course of a therapeutic hour. I frequently use games and drawing, both of which rapidly absorb attention and can provide a transition to hypnosis.

Dr. Valerie Wall (1988) underscores the need for non-authoritarian and permissive inductions, which allow for maximum interaction with the therapist. Dr. Marlene Hunter (1994) points out that it is common for children to be engaged in trance with their eyes open and with considerable physical movement. In my (GG) own experience using Arm Catalepsy (see Chapter 5) with children, I have noticed that they commonly giggle and fidget while watching their arm first float and then sink down to the comfort of their lap. Hunter (1994) adds that children are highly resourceful and that, as we are telling them a story, they will often be far ahead of us, eager to supply their own conclusion without our having to do so for them. The resources of children are different from those of adults, but rich and abundant just the same. These resources may be nothing more than their imaginations or a restless activity that can be utilized to induce trance.

In the Family Therapy Training Program at the Tucson V.A. we primarily treat children within the context of marital and family problems, and the two inductions that follow are examples of a wide array of inductions useful in an office-based practice. Olness and Kohen's (1996) *Hypnosis and Hypnotherapy with Children (Third Edition)*, remains required reading for those who wish to explore this topic further. Their list of age-appropriate induction techniqes is included as Table 6.1. This table offers a variety of induction techniques for children of all ages. Storytelling, Favorite Place, and Favorite Activity are usually the inductions of choice with most children over age four.

In working with children as well as adults, we rely heavily on therapeutic stories. We use stories in books, such as Nancy Davis's (1990) *Therapeutic Stories to Heal Abused Children*. Stories with specific applications, such as those in Davis's book, can be adapted for other problems. We have stock stories, but we also make up stories in the middle of a session. This process need not be long or complex. It may simply involve an example of another child. "Let me tell you a story about someone else just about your age. . . ." Start out the story by *pacing* or modeling the client's world, which shows that you understand, e.g., "She also had a brother and a sister and her parents were divorced . . . ," and then *lead*, or add on, in the desired direction, e.g., ". . . and she discovered *one thing* that really helped her at school as well as at home. . . ."

We often tell the story of Pandora's box during the first session with children age seven and older. You may remember this ancient Greek tale about a young girl named Pandora. The gods give her a heavy, jewel-encrusted box along with instructions to *never open* the box. With the passage of time, Pandora's curiosity gets the best of her. She pries the box open, and all the evils of the world fly out. (We like to update the tale by saying things like, ". . . and all the evils of the world flew out of the box: sadness, divorce, AIDS . . ."). Then Pandora sees something gleaming down in the bottom of the box. It is hope. An important meta-message in this story is that self-disclosure is okay.

When we see children in therapy (whether or not we are doing hypnosis) we always have food available. Cookies, pretzels, or similar snacks help break the ice and warm them to therapy. Children, like adults, may harbor negative misconceptions about hypnosis, and some believe that in trance they may fall asleep or lose control. It is important to address these issues in pre-trance discussion. Also, we always gain parental consent before commencing treatment.

TABLE 6.1 Induction Techniques by Age

Preverbal (0–2 years)

Tactile stimulation, stroking, patting
Kinesthetic stimulation: rocking,
    moving an arm back and forth
Auditory stimulation: music or any
    whirring sound such as a hairdryer,
    electric shaver, vacuum cleaner
    placed out of reach of the child
Visual stimulation: mobiles or other
    objects that change shape, color, or
    position
Holding a doll or stuffed animal

Early verbal (2–4 years)

Blowing bubbles
Pop-up books
Storytelling
Stereoscopic viewer
Favorite activity
Speaking to the child through a doll or
    stuffed animal
Floppy Raggedy Ann or Andy
Teddy bear
Watching induction or self on videotape

Preschool and early school (4–6 years)

Blowing breath out
Favorite place
Multiple animals
Flower garden
Storytelling (alone or in a group)
Mighty oak tree
Coin watching
Letter watching
Pop-up books
Television fantasy
Stereoscopic viewer
Videotape
Bouncing ball
Thermal (and other) biofeedback
Finger lowering
Playground activity

Middle childhood (7–11 years)

Favorite place
Favorite activity
Cloud gazing
Flying blanket
Videogames (actual or imagined)
Riding a bike
Arm lowering
Blowing breath out
Favorite music
Listening to self on tape
Coin watching
Fixation at point on hand
Hands (fingers) moving together
Arm rigidity

Adolescence (12–18 years)

Favorite place/activity
Sports activity
Arm catalepsy
Following breathing
Videogames (actual or imagined)
Computer games (actual or imag-
    ined)
Eye fixation on hand
Driving a car
Playing or hearing music
Hand levitation
Fingers / hands together as
    magnets
Fantasy games (e.g., Dungeons
    and Dragons)

From Olness and Kohen (1996). Reprinted with permission from Guilford.

UTILIZATION

Carlos, age six, was a bully to classmates at school and to his four-year-old sister at home. His parents, who unexpectedly brought him along for their third session of marital therapy, indicated that the boy was scheduled to be evaluated by the school psychologist in three weeks. The couple blamed Carlos for their unhappiness. "Please do something with this boy," they insisted.

Carlos wore Army fatigues identical to those worn by his father, also named Carlos, a poorly adjusted Latino Vietnam veteran, age 45, who was now married to Maria, a woman from Mexico who spoke little English. Maria was his fifth wife, the mother of Carlos and his sister. It was no surprise that little Carlos was trying to survive the best he could in a chaotic and highly dysfunctional family.

An available intern saw little Carlos while we resumed marital therapy. The intern learned that in addition to Nintendo and watching cartoons, Carlos's favorite activity was *marching in place*. The boy demonstrated how he marched "just like Dad" did, through the jungles of Southeast Asia. Carlos would pause now and then to shoot an imaginary enemy, tiger, or snake. Carlos said yes when asked if he would like to learn how to relax so that he could march even better. The boy, who was cooperative and appeared to be of average intelligence, had heard of hypnosis but did not really know what it was. Carlos was adept at *marching in place*, and would do so immediately when requested. The next day we were able to recreate the essentials of the induction.

Induction

Carlos, keep marching in place just like you're doing, at a nice easy pace, *one foot down* and then *the other foot up, down and up*, feeling that floor underneath your feet, and *arms moving* at your side, *and* no doubt you can *imagine*, Carlos, *just imagine*, where you are right now, pretending, in your mind, and tell me, Carlos, where are you?

    ("Vietnam," he answers.)

pacing

linking word
leading

And this Vietnam, I wonder what
it is . . . .

("It's a place with a big jungle. Lots
of enemies." He pauses to shoot one.
"Bang! Yer dead. I won't cut off yer ears
this time, enemy, 'cause I already got a
whole string of ears around my neck.
Bang! Another one's dead!")

Just keep marching, Carlos, nice and
easy, and *I wonder when* my words will   *implication*
begin to drift in, or drift out of your
ears, your own ears, Carlos, that's the
way . . .

By the way, Carlos, where is this
Vietnam?

("Close to New York," he answers.)

And now *I wonder when those feet*   *implication*
will feel like marching faster, *all by*
themselves, faster . . . and still a bit   *involuntariness*
faster yet . . .

(Carlos quickens his pace.)

. . . and faster, so that you start to
breathe hard, *and* as you do that, *you*   *linking word*
will find that it's not necessary to shoot   *contingent suggestion*
your gun anymore because you won't be
seeing any more "enemies," is that
okay with you?

("Sure," he says, and he is panting
now.)

And now I'd like you to really *slow*   *suggestion*
down your marching, nice and slow,
kind of like *seeing a boy on TV*, march-   *metaphor*
ing in slow motion, *slow motion on TV*,
and you can *see* that boy, or *imagine*   *bind of comparable*
him, or actually *picture* him on TV,   *alternatives*
huh?

(Carlos nods.)

As you slow down, slowing way   *contingent suggestion*

down, those feet may *begin to feel* very, very heavy, like you have big cowboy boots on those feet . . .

("Army boots—these are army boots," he says, as he points to his tennis shoes.)

And with *those* feet feeling so very heavy, the *rest of your body can also feel heavy and slowed down . . . and so, too, with your mind,* just like slow motion on TV, that's the way . . .

dissociation

contingent suggestions

Carlos, whenever you need to slow down your mind, and slow down your body, you can march real slowly like this. . . . I *wonder*, and I also *imagine* if there are times at home, or at school, when you feel angry, or upset . . .

hypnotic language

("When Mom yells at me," he exclaims)

What about at school?

("I hate school," he says.)

You did a real good job marching in place here today, Carlos, and I would like you to come back here another day and do the same thing. How about that?

("Sure," he says.)

And just *standing there* like that, in that same place, and *starting to move your feet*, that can be a signal to you to begin to slow down and relax.

posthypnotic suggestion

Deepening

No deepening was done during this rather brief, impromptu session. For subsequent sessions we used descending a staircase.

REALERTING

Carlos was instructed to stop moving his feet and to simply sit down in an adjacent chair. He quickly realerted.

DEBRIEFING

Usually with younger children it is not necessary to spend as much time as you would with adolescents or adults ratifying trance. Time distortion, amnesia, and ideosensory feeling are abstract concepts. Instead, they see trance as a game. Carlos was praised for doing a good job.

NOTES FOR PRACTICE

Our goal for Carlos was essentially to help him be less of a bully by teaching him to manage stress, which he did with three more sessions of therapy. In working with highly dysfunctional families, the real work is with the parents; however, in working with parents who are child-focused (*"Do* something with this kid!"), it is important to not ignore their request or else they may drop out of therapy.

Carlos never did receive an evaluation from the school psychologist because the parents failed to keep the appointment. Shortly after beginning treatment Carlos, Sr., was arrested for driving under the influence and received court-ordered substance abuse treatment. This was followed by a three-month intensive inpatient PTSD treatment at another V.A. The parents then did well with several sessions of marital therapy with a focus on parenting. Although the family remained dysfunctional, they eventually achieved a modicum of stability. Both Carlos and his father discarded their army fatigues and began to wear conventional clothing. At last report Carlos was no longer marching, but he was moving his feet fast in a youth soccer league.

Some may find it repellent to engage a young child around militaristic behavior that includes atrocities such as taking ears from dead enemies. Whether or not the father actually did these things, we will never know. The important thing is that this behavior was present in a family with nonexistent boundaries. The behavior, however distasteful, is part of the total package that the client brings to therapy. First it must be accepted and embraced—all of it—and then it can be utilized.

MY FRIEND JOHN

In the family therapy training program at the Tucson V.A. we commonly see adolescents who present with symptoms associated with marital or family discord. Many of these young people are interested in hypnosis and will respond favorably to straightforward inductions. With adolescents, it is important to spend a session or two connecting with their pain, confusion, or isolation. This is especially true for teenagers experiencing separation, divorce, or stepfamily problems.

The My Friend John technique is one that we use occasionally with adults, but more frequently with adolescents. Erickson named and popularized this technique (Rossi, 1980) for use with highly resistant clients who had no interest in hypnosis but agreed to Erickson's hypnotizing an imaginary person, "my friend John." With this by proxy induction it is often difficult for the client to not self-reference or incorporate the suggestions directed at the imaginary person.

Shawnee is a 13-year-old girl who grew up in Colorado and was adopted at age two by a couple we were seeing for marital therapy. The couple asked us to see Shawnee because of her rebelliousness, defiance, and poor grades in school, the onset of which corresponded with the beginning of marital conflict two years previously. Shawnee bristled with anger and provided minimal answers to general questions directed at getting to know her. We immediately decided to try to discharge resistance by two techniques. The first one involved asking her to change chairs, which she did, the idea being that some of her resistance would be left in the first chair. The second technique involved asking a series of questions to which she had to answer no. It is presumed that negativity is discharged with each no response.

"Shawnee, do you like being here today?"
"No."
"And I'm safe to assume that you like me?"
"No."
"And I suppose you like everybody at school?"
"No."
"Then you hate everybody at school, and you don't have any friends at all, right?"
"No."
"So, is there one person at school you dislike more than everybody else? A teacher, another student?"
"Mrs. Cornelius I don't like. She's a teacher. Dori I like.She's a student."

"Shawnee, for my own amusement, or maybe for some other reason that will become apparent later, I would like to hypnotize an imaginary girl over there in that chair. Let's call her Dori. You mind if I do that?"

"Knock yourself out."

"Okay, and while I do this you can just sit there and pay attention if you want, or just disregard the whole thing. Another girl just about your age, Anne, who moved here from Chicago—not from Colorado—she sat there and tried very hard to block out everything, and we can only imagine how well she did doing precisely that."

Induction

Dori, I know that you *came some distance* over here today, driving *in your parents' car across town, braving the windstorm* that we had earlier in the afternoon, and then *coming in here, sitting down there*, first in one chair, and then another, and I know, and you might already guess that you can go into trance just as deeply as you want, recognizing that a person has many options, being able to choose between a *light trance, medium trance, or deep trance*, which can be a very pleasant and comfortable experience.

(Casually observing Shawnee) Dori, *looking around the room, and moving around in your chair*, no doubt the *intensity of feeling* you're experiencing can propel you *strongly, convincingly, or forcefully* into a pleasant state of relaxation, but *no one should ever let go too fast*, Dori, *and* you might find that it's comfortable to *let your eyes settle on just one thing* in this room—*or maybe something else over there*—and you might know from experience that

truisms

*bind of comparable
alternatives*

pacing

*reframe
bind of comparable
alternatives
restraint
linking word
suggestion*

pacing

looking at one spot for a long time is something that a person can become *absorbed in*, or *immersed in*, or maybe it's being *pleasantly distracted*, I don't know, kind of like at home, Dori, or at school, when something catches your attention and you *stay with it, just staying with it* . . . and then *time*, as we know it, on a watch or on a clock, can seem to really *slow down*, or maybe it *speeds up*, or maybe it *doesn't really matter at all what a person does, or thinks*, and with all this interesting stuff going on *outside* a person can begin to slow down on the *inside* and notice particular feelings in her body, *wondering when* will a *lightness* or *heaviness* or *tingling* or *numbness* or some other interesting sensation begin to *develop and spread out, slowing down her mind and her body, and* a person's eyes *eventually feel tired and blink . . . and then blink again and then her breathing* can become more and more regular, slowed down, *and* if those eyes want to gently close on their own, they may, or else just keep looking at that spot is fine, too.

bind of comparable alternatives

suggestion

time distortion

not knowing/not doing

apposition of opposites

implication

apposition of opposites
implication
linking word
implication
pacing
leading
linking word

Deepening

I bet you never thought you could go deeper into trance by breaking rocks, yes, I said breaking rocks. Now I'd like you to imagine you're outside somewhere, it's daytime, and you're standing in front of a huge pile of rocks, a mountain of rocks.

(Shawnee maintains eye fixation on the wall. She sighs deeply, but nonverbally betrays neither agreement nor rejection of the image put forth so far.)

There is a path leading up to the pile of rocks, and in your mind, I'd like you to walk up to the top of the pile, taking as much time as you need. That's the way, Dori. Up there at the top you will find a sledge hammer, one that you can easily pick up, and there's also a pair of goggles that you can put on because we know what it's like when rocks are smashed into lots of small pieces. Now, Dori, in your mind, I'd like you to pick up that sledge hammer and start smashing those rocks, pounding them, breaking them, one after another, just releasing all those strong, pent-up feelings each time you break a rock. You keep smashing those rocks until you're exhausted, letting go of all those strong, strong feelings. That's the way. . . .

(Shawnee remains focused on a spot on the wall. She is breathing faster now. Her right hand is grasping her thigh.)

And any time in the future when you feel the need to let go of strong feelings, all you have to do is just reach down and grab your thigh, just squeezing like that . . .

(She immediately relaxes her right hand and rolls it into a fist.)

REALERTING

We realert the client with the following: "Dori, in a moment I'm going to have you wake up, and anyone else in the room who feels like waking up can just stop looking at the wall, and be ready to take a guess at how much time passed here today."

DEBRIEFING

Shawnee ceased eye fixation, glared at me and said, "You didn't fool me any. I knew what you were doing all the time." "You looked pretty relaxed," I ventured. "I was bored, that's all," she said. "You're a very boring man." "I've had to work hard for many years to be good at being boring," I admitted.

NOTES FOR PRACTICE

Shawnee reluctantly returned with her parents five more times. By the third session she said it was okay to say her name instead of Dori's. She then closed her eyes and went into trance quite readily with a conversational induction. She never did admit that trancework helped her and said that she was just going along with it to help her parents, who reported an improvement in her behavior at school and at home. I maintained a posture of restraint with Shawnee, praising her effort while at the same time admitting that my telling her stories about other girls and boys who overcame adversity would probably do no good at all. I never knew what worked in this case—whether it was hypnotherapy with Shawnee, simultaneous gains in marital therapy, or a little of both.

We use the pile of rocks as an intervention technique for anger and anxiety. It is directive but also permissive in that clients fill in the details. I (GG) first heard of this in 1994 from Dr. Claire Frederick when she presented a workshop at an American Society of Clinical Hypnosis training in California. It is usually employed as a highly interactive technique in that, at each step along the way, you ask for a response from the client, verifying that they have walked up to the top of the pile, for example. At the end, an anchor such as a fist or a deep breath is installed. This technique was used as a deepening with Shawnee in order to begin to address her anger. Employed indirectly in this way, it allowed her to self-reference the metaphor.

Glossary

abreaction Trauma clients may experience intense emotions such as panic or fear, which may be accompanied by flashbacks or intrusive thoughts. This expression of emotions may occur not only during direct treatment of the trauma, but also during simple relaxation. In hypnotherapy, one of several techniques for treating trauma involves age regression to a time the trauma occurred, a facilitated abreaction, and reframing. This process often provides the client considerable relief and a new understanding of the traumatic experience. This should be attempted only by experienced therapists. Incomplete abreaction of underlying feelings may be a cause of therapeutic failure.

absorption of attention Necessary for successful trance, the client's attention is focused on, for example, a spot on the wall, a story, a bodily sensation, or anything else. Eye fixation, eye closure, facial mask, diminished movement, lack of swallowing, and other signs may indicate an absorption of attention.

age progression Essentially the opposite of age regression, clients are asked to imagine themselves in the future, feeling or behaving confident, strong, or in control. The technique is also called time projection, among other names.

age regression A technique useful in hypnotherapy for accessing resources during problem solving and other applications, age regression is experienced naturally whenever someone has a memory or reminiscence. As part of trancework, age regression may be structured and guided, e.g., "I want you to ride a magic carpet back through time to age 15," or general and permissive, e.g., "I want you, starting now, to go back in your own way, taking as much time as you need, back to any time in the past that might be important to the problem at hand, and when you get there, let me know by nodding your head. . . ." We should try not to impede clients, as they invariably go back in time much faster than we can guide them.

amnesia Some practitioners believe that inducing amnesia is necessary for later problem resolution, as amnesia allows unconscious processing to go on without conscious interference. Amnesia can be encouraged with suggestions such as "Will you forget to remember, or simply remember to forget?" or "When you go to sleep you dream, and when you wake up you cannot remember that dream." Many clients will have amnesia for some portion of the trance experience even if it is not facilitated.

and A very important word in psychotherapy, *and* leads and links. Following a pacing statement, e.g., "You feel the comfort of that one deep breath," the word then leads, "*and* you can use that one deep breath to let yourself sink deeper and deeper. . . ." It may also link a truism to a directive or suggestion, e.g., "You have experienced the comfort of trance here for the past 30 minutes or so, *and* you can now begin to use this experience at work when you need it the most. . . ."

apposition of opposites An example of hypnotic language, this technique juxtaposes polarities or opposites, e.g., "As that right hand develops a *lightness*, your body can sink even deeper into *heaviness* and relaxation." The therapist can experiment with warm-cold, up-down, light-heavy, right-left, or any number of opposites.

arm catalepsy Catalepsy means a suspension of movement. In this book, a cataleptic or rigid arm is part of the Arm Catalepsy induction, an effective, rapid, and highly directive means for inducing trance.

bind of comparable alternatives A potent ally of the therapist, this appears to offer the client a choice between two or more alternatives, offering the illusion of choice, e.g., "Today would you like to go into a light trance, a medium trance, or a deep trance?" or "What you learned today might be useful in your personal life, or maybe you can use it at work, or perhaps you can simply incorporate it into your overall experience."

commitment Social psychology ascertains that if people commit to doing something, they are more likely to comply. A vital concept in hypnotherapy, commitment is a potent therapeutic tool for increasing the effectiveness of suggestions, e.g., "Taking one deep breath can help you in a stressful situation. If this is something you're willing to practice at least once a day, your *yes* finger will rise." (See also **unconscious commitment**.)

confusion Employed to counter unconscious resistance, this is a broad category of techniques that interrupt, overload, or distract the conscious mind. In this book, the non sequitur is used, e.g., "I wonder why shopping carts always seem to stick together," and as the client tries to make sense of the confusing statement, she is receptive to a suggestion, e.g., "You can go deep," an avenue of escape provided by the therapist. Confusion is generally more effective in short bursts, and should always be used judiciously and respectfully.

conscious-unconscious bind A bind limits choice, channeling behavior in the desired direction. This type of suggestion helps bypass conscious, learned limitations by accessing the unconscious mind, e.g., "An unconscious learning from this experience today may be developed in your conscious mind as well" or "When your conscious mind is ready to provide some useful information about this problem, you will experience a peculiar sensation in your right hand. If such information comes from your unconscious mind, the sensation will be in your left hand."

contingent suggestion Also known as chaining, this type of suggestion connects the suggestion to an ongoing or inevitable behavior, e.g., "And as you become aware of that peculiar sensation in your right hand, you can begin to float back in time"; or as a posthypnotic suggestion, "When you return here and sit there in that chair, you can resume that deep and pleasant sense of relaxation." It is believed that it is more difficult to reject two or more suggestions when they are linked together in this way.

displacement As used for pain management, the locus of pain is displaced to another area of the body or to an area outside the body. The client may continue to experience the sensation, but in a less painful or vulnerable way.

dissociative language Dissociation is a hallmark of trance and an excellent convincer of trance. The more clients experience it, e.g., their hand separated from their body, the more their hypnotic experience is ratified. Whenever possible, the therapist should say *that* hand instead of *your* hand, and employ similar language, especially during induction and deepening. Encouraging dissociation deepens trance.

double dissociative conscious-unconscious double bind Confusional suggestions such as this are complex and interesting. However, they are probably the least important type of suggestion to become skillful in using. Example: "Between now and next time your conscious mind may work at resolving the problem while your unconscious mind wonders about the implications, or your unconscious mind may come up with answers while your unconscious mind ponders the implications."

double negative An example of hypnotic language, it is believed that a double negative may lead some clients to accept the suggestion more than a simple positive suggestion alone. For example, "You can't not pay attention to the warmth developing in the soles of your feet." The two negatives negate each other to form a positive suggestion, and the hint of confusion enhances acceptance. (See also **triple negative**.)

embedded suggestion The client's conscious mind is bypassed when the therapist embeds a suggestion. To encourage an inward focus, the therapist may embed *in* words, e.g., "Going *in*side can be very *int*eresting . . . *in* there where you have your imagi*n*ation, fasci-*n*ation, *int*uition. . . ." Also, the therapist might suggest *security*, for example, by embedding it in a story that emphasizes *security* provided at a large outdoor concert.

eye closure   Some therapists feel uncomfortable if clients do not readily close their eyes. We can suggest that their eyes will blink, their eyelids might feel heavy, and that their eyes can gently close whenever they wish. Clients can experience deep trance through eye fixation alone, and open eyes permit the therapist an observation of ongoing process.

eye fixation   For clients who fear loss of control, it is helpful to let them focus their gaze on a spot of their choice, e.g., somewhere on the wall, the ceiling, or the back of their hand. They may eventually feel comfortable enough to close their eyes.

fluff   This refers to meaningless filler that the therapist includes either in the conversational patter in an induction, or in a story. Purposeless, meandering detail is thought to bore the client and deepen absorption. A therapist we work with once said, "It took many years for me to learn to be boring." Too often we may believe that things we say to the client must be purposeful or didactic; however, a few well-placed suggestions inserted amidst a flurry of fluff may be much more effective.

hypnotic language   Certain words such as *story, imagine, wonder, curious, explore,* and *interesting* are thought to activate a sense of wonderment, which may enhance the trance process.

implication   An important method of indirect suggestion, the therapist stimulates trance experience by conveying positive expectancy. "When you are aware of warmth beginning to spread out, you may nod your head." The therapist does not ask, "*Does* one of your hands feel *light*?" but, "*Which* one of your hands is *lighter*?" In implication, *when* is often the operative word, not the authoritarian *will*, which does not imply or suggest, but commands or directs. In accessing unconscious resources, the therapist may say, "Taking as much time as you need, *when* your unconscious mind has selected some strength or resource from the past, your yes finger can move all by itself."

interspersal　The therapist's hypnotic patter is interspersed with words, phrases, metaphors, or anecdotes to indirectly influence the client. For example, while therapists count backward from ten to one during deepening, they may insert a brief anecdote about another client who experienced a peculiar heaviness in her hand. Words such as *heavy, light,* or *deep* or a phrase such as "Just let go" may be inserted randomly. Attention is drawn to an interspersed suggestion that is set apart from hypnotic patter by a pause, and thus it becomes more potent.

issues of control and trust　Clients need to be reassured that they will not lose control during the session. Building rapport and trust neutralizes this fear, as does concrete reassurance, e.g., "You are always in the driver's seat," or perhaps humorously, "Don't worry, I'll tell you if you quack like a duck." Trust is also maintained by discussing the agenda for the session. For example, we would not want to do age regression without permission.

law of parsimony　This "law" holds that the therapist should say or do as little as is necessary to achieve the desired response. A long or elaborate induction is not necessary if the client can go into trance by simply recalling a pleasant scene. With a client experienced in trancework, this less-is-more approach is manifested by a minimalist induction such as "Just sit back now, close your eyes, and let yourself go into trance."

metaphor　A broad class of indirect techniques, the use of metaphor allows the therapist to bypass the conscious mind and tap into unconscious processes, which tend to be represented and comprehended metaphorically. A client's situation or idiosyncratic speech, such as "I feel like there is a wall around me," provides the therapist with imagery to be utilized. Stories or symbols stimulate self-referencing at an unconscious level.

naturalistic trance states　Pre-hypnosis discussion should elicit situations when the client naturally drifts off or becomes absorbed in something pleasant, such as a favorite activity. This establishes trance as a naturally occurring behavior within the client's control. Examples include "highway hypnosis" while driving, immersion in a book or movie, etc.

negative hallucination Milton Erickson employed *positive* hallucination when he had children imagine a furry animal next to them. Even more useful—and easier to induce—is negative hallucination, e.g., "You will notice the sound of the air conditioner, people talking in the hallway, and my voice speaking to you, and all these sounds may simply drift in and out of your ears, or you may not hear them at all."

negative reframe To be used judiciously, a negative reframe is useful for redirecting the client's attention or perturbing monolithic behavior. A man's reluctance to carry out an assignment can be reframed as passivity or weakness. A woman's interpersonal conflict can be reframed as uncaring or unprotective.

non sequitur Used for distraction or interruption, a statement that is totally out of context can depotentiate conscious mental sets. One of a wide variety of confusion techniques such as statements or stories, a non sequitur can overload or distract the conscious mind. As the conscious mind seeks to escape from this incongruence or dissonance, the client may be receptive to suggestion, e.g., an ego-strengthening suggestion, "You can do it." Non sequiturs can be virtually any phrase or question, e.g., "And the rain fell silently in the forest" or "Do you like dogs?"

not knowing/not doing Actually a suggestion for restraint, this elegant device is very liberating in that it facilitates unconscious responsiveness rather than conscious effort. The therapeutic process may be facilitated if, early in the induction, the therapist says something like, "There's absolutely nothing to do, or to know, or to think about, or to change; in fact, isn't it nice to know that by just sitting there and breathing, you can go into trance, and you don't even have to listen to the words." It may also help clients discharge resistance or anxiety.

permissive suggestion It is believed that many clients respond well when given a wide range of choice, e.g., "You may begin to notice sensations, feelings, or experiences beginning to develop in those hands, or will it be in your feet?"

positive expectancy Clients are more likely to be responsive when the therapist conveys confidence and certainty that improvement can be expected. The therapist may express confidence or hopefulness about a successful problem resolution, or during an induction, when the therapist suggests hand levitation, both his verbal and nonverbal behavior convey overt positive expectancy.

posthypnotic suggestion This is a suggestion, given in trance, for behavior to occur outside of trance. For example, "When you return here next time and sit down there, the feeling of that chair will be a signal for you to resume the pleasantness and relaxation of trance" or, "At work or at home you will be able to begin to relax when you take one big, deep satisfying breath" or, "During the next two weeks when you're going to work on the bus and you cross 22nd Street you will notice something that can help you with this problem. . . ." The last posthypnotic suggestion—notice something—is tagged to a naturally occurring behavior.

pun A play on words can cause a sense of wonderment. An embedded suggestion in a pun is a useful indirect technique, e.g., "Your experience in trance today is like an *entrance* into another state."

question A direct question will focus attention, stimulate associations, and facilitate responsiveness. A question such as "And the tingling down there in that foot, do you notice it yet?" bypasses the conscious mind and is useful as a probe when the therapist is discovering the client's hypnotic talents, or when resistance is present.

reframe A new understanding or appreciation comes about because of new information provided by the therapist. By relabeling or wrapping a positive connotation around problem behavior, the client is given hope, along with seeing the problem in a new light. Virtually anything the client brings to therapy may be reframed. The session itself may be reframed as an effort to make things better. When there is little to reframe, therapists may reframe the presumed motivation *behind* the distress or problem in the same way that they may reframe the therapy session itself as an *effort*, or *intention*, to make things better. A reframe also sets the stage for a suggestion or directive, so that it is more likely to be accepted. Reframe is a vital element in all methods of psychotherapy, as virtually any behavior can be reframed as strength, protectiveness, caring, or any other value dear to the client. (See also **negative reframe**.)

repetition Suggestions that are important should be repeated. The therapist may repeat "breathing in comfort and relaxation" several times in an induction. It is also useful to repeat a suggestion in a different way, e.g., "feeling a particular heaviness in those feet" may be followed later by the same suggestion that is metaphorical: "Another person felt like he had heavy boots on his feet, and he could barely move them."

resistance A client who says, "I don't want to go into trance" displays conscious resistance. A client who says, "I want to go into trance, but I just can't" is showing unconscious resistance. Many clients are keenly aware of their resistance, which may be anxiety, negativity, or feared loss of control. Resistance may be discharged in various ways, including general and permissive suggestions, suggestions covering all possibilities, not knowing/not doing, metaphor, story, confusion techniques, having the client switch chairs (so he leaves his resistance in the first chair), and asking the client questions to which he must answer no, e.g., "In the winter the temperature in Phoenix is the same as in Minneapolis." Many times clients' resistance will abate as rapport builds, and as they feel more comfortable in therapy.

restraint Resistant clients may become more resistant if we encourage change or adaptation too rapidly. These clients' resistance can be lessened if we restrain or hold them back from moving ahead, e.g., "Go slow . . . change presents uncertainty . . . you might not be ready yet . . . it could be dangerous to move ahead too fast." Early in trancework, inducing trance, bringing clients out of trance, and then resuming hypnosis, holds back something pleasant, builds responsiveness, and enhances client control.

seeding A suggestion may be more successful when it has been mentioned, or seeded, beforehand. A target suggestion is seeded, and later, mentioning the suggestion again, the target is activated. In prehypnosis, the therapist may mention breathing, slowing down, or deep relaxation, as these suggestions will follow in trancework. If therapists know that they will be offering suggestions to slow down eating, they can cue this idea by appreciably slowing down their rhythm in advance.

speaking the client's language By incorporating the client's own language, literally using the words of the client, the therapist's suggestions may conform more to the client's thinking and be more effective.

suggestion covering all possibilities This can be especially useful when combined with metaphor, e.g., describing someone else's experience in trance: "As a person goes deeper into trance she can begin to notice various sensations starting to develop in her hands. It might be a tingling in one hand; maybe a numbness in the other; perhaps a warm feeling, or a cold one, or some other interesting feeling. One woman one time sitting right there in that chair wondered privately, 'How is it that one time coming in here I can sense a slight coldness up here in my right ear lobe, and another time I feel a tingling down there in my right big toe?'" (See also **bind of comparable alternatives** and **permissive suggestion**.)

time distortion This is a common trance phenomenon, as time may seem to speed up or slow down during trance. "How much time do you think has passed since you came in here?" is a relevant question to ask clients when they come out of trance. This ratifies the trance experience and is an indicator of responsiveness.

triple negative It is believed that a triple negative is received positively by the unconscious mind. A statement such as "Your unconscious mind *never can't not* process this problem between now and next session" may facilitate processing, or it might best serve to give the client a mild confusion or pleasant sense of wonderment.

truism This is an undeniable statement of fact, e.g., "Everyone has felt the warm sun on their skin." A series of truisms leads to a yes-set that builds commitment and acceptance of ideas, e.g., "Coming in here today on a hot day, sitting for a while out there in the waiting room, walking down the hall, coming in here, and sitting down there, I know that you can begin to let yourself go. . . ." (See also **yes-set**.)

unconscious commitment Therapists may consult the unconscious mind through nonverbal signalling, e.g., "And when your unconscious mind has identified a time in the past when you felt confident, you may signal with your yes finger." Unconscious commitment is obtained by a direct question, e.g., "I want to direct a question to your unconscious mind: After exploring this problem and understanding it as you do, are you now willing to let go of the problem? Taking as much time as you need, you may signal with one of your fingers." (See also **commitment**.)

unconscious mind Many writers refer to this construct as meaning virtually any thought or feeling that is outside of the client's immediate awareness. With some clients, it may be helpful to refer to this as either "the subsconscious mind" or "the back part of the mind."

utilization Tailoring therapy, or hypnosis, to the individual takes into account the client's unique motivations, interests, preferences, and use of language. The client's behavior, however problematic, is accepted and suggestions are attached to it, e.g., the client yawns and the therapist notes, "Have you ever noticed how even a simple yawn can lead to even deeper relaxation?" The therapist conveys the importance of utterly accepting whatever occurs with the client and then seeks to use and transform it. The therapist follows and then guides the ongoing behavior of the client.

yes-set An ally of the therapist in any modality, this involves mentioning truisms, or aspects of undeniable reality, to create a "yes-set" acceptance, thus allowing the client to be more receptive to a suggestion that follows. For example, "You've done very well coming in here for five sessions now, working hard each time, *and* I know that today you can make even more progress toward your goal."

Hypnosis Organizations

The American Society of Clinical Hypnosis (ASCH), 33 W. Grand Avenue, Suite 402, Chicago, Illinois 60610. Tel: 312-645-9810, fax: 312-645-9818. Several times a year ASCH provides regional workshops in the U.S. on clinical hypnosis. Members receive *The American Journal of Clinical Hypnosis*. ASCH Press has various publications available. In addition to membership, ASCH provides a certification in clinical hypnosis and an approved consultant certification.

The Milton H. Erickson Foundation, 3606 N. 24th Street, Phoenix, Arizona 85016. Tel: 602-956-6196, fax: 602-956-0519, e-mail: office@ erickson-foundation.org (http://www.erickson-foundation.org). The Erickson Foundation provides a variety of training in the U.S. and other countries. Members receive the *Newsletter of the Milton H. Erickson Foundation*. The Erickson Foundation has many component organizations in the U.S. and other countries.

The Society for Clinical and Experimental Hypnosis (SCEH), 2201 Haeder Road, Pullman, WA 99163. Tel: 509-332-7555, fax: 509-332-5907, e-mail: sceh@pullman.com. SCEH provides training opportunities along with other services and publishes the *International Journal of Clinical and Experimental Hypnosis*.

References

American Society of Clinical Hypnosis Committee on Hypnosis and Memory Report (1995). *Clinical hypnosis and memory: Guidelines for clinicians and for forensic hypnosis*. Chicago: American Society of Clinical Hypnosis.

Araoz, D. L. (1985). *The new hypnosis*. New York: Brunner/Mazel.

Bandler, R., & Grinder, J. (1982.) *Reframing: Neuro-linguistic programming and the transformation of meaning*. Moab, UT: Real People.

Barber, J. (1996). *Hypnosis and suggestion in the treatment of pain*. New York: Norton.

Beahrs, J. O. (1971). The hypnotic psychotherapy of Milton H. Erickson. *American Journal of Clinical Hypnosis*, *14*(3), 73–90.

Bird, N. (1997.) Treatment of dental phobia using a modified television visualization technique. *Contemporary Hypnosis*, *14*(1), 80–83.

Cheek, D. (1994). *Hypnosis: The application of ideomotor techniques.* Needham Heights, MA: Allyn & Bacon.

Citrenbaum, C. M., King, M. E., & Cohen, W. I. (1985). *Modern clinical hypnosis for habit control.* New York: Norton.

Combs, G., & Freedman, J. (1990). *Symbol, story, and ceremony: Using metaphor in individual and family therapy.* New York: Norton.

Crasilneck, H. B. (1982). A follow-up study in the use of hypnotherapy in the treatment of psychogenic impotence. *American Journal of Clinical Hypnosis, 25*(1), 52–61.

Crasilneck, H. B., & Hall, J. A. (1985). *Clinical hypnosis: Principles and applications.* Orlando, FL: Grune & Stratton.

Davis, N. (1990). *Therapeutic stories to heal abused children.* Oxenhill, MD: Psychosocial Associates.

Dahlgren, L. A., Jurtz, R. M., Strube, M. J., & Malone, M. D. (1995). Differential effects of hypnotic suggestion on multiple dimensions of pain. *Journal of Pain Symptom Management, 10*(6), 464–470.

Dolan, Y. (1991). *Resolving sexual abuse.* New York: Norton.

Erickson, M. H., Rossi, E. I., & Rossi, S. I. (1976). *Hypnotic realities.* New York: Irvington.

Felt, B. T., Hall, H., Olness, K., Schmidt, W., Kohen, D., Berman, B. D., Broffman, G., Coury, D., French, G., Dattner, A., & Young, M. H. (1998). Wart regression in children: Comparison of relaxation-imagery to topical treatment and equal time interventions. *American Journal of Clinical Hypnosis, 41*(2), 130–137.

Fischman, Y. (1991). Interacting with trauma: Clinicians' responses to treating psychological aftereffects of political repression. *American Journal of Orthopsychiatry, 61*(2), 179–185.

Gafner, G. (1997). Hypnotherapy with older adults. *Contemporary Hypnosis, 14*(1), 68–79.

Gafner, G., & Duckett, S. (1992). Treating the sequelae of a curse in elderly Mexican-Americans. In T. L. Brink (Ed.), *Hispanic aged mental health* (pp. 45–53). New York: Haworth.

Gafner, G., & Young, C. (1998). Hypnosis as an adjuvant treatment in chronic paranoid schizophrenia. *Contemporary Hypnosis, 15*(4), 223–226.

Geary, B. (1994). Seeding responsiveness to hypnotic processes. In J. K. Zeig (Ed.), *Ericksonian methods* (pp. 315–332). New York: Brunner/Mazel.

Gilligan, S. (1987). *Therapeutic trances: The cooperation principle in Ericksonian hypnotherapy*. New York: Brunner/Mazel.

Haley, J. (1973). *Uncommon therapy: The psychiatric techniques of Milton H. Erickson, M.D.* New York: Norton.

Hammond, D. C. (1988). *Hypnotic induction and suggestion: An introductory manual*. Des Plaines, IL: American Society of Clinical Hypnosis.

Hammond, D. C. (1990). *Handbook of hypnotic suggestions and metaphors*. New York: Norton.

Hartland, H. E. (1971). Further observations on the use of ego-strengthening techniques. *American Journal of Clinical Hypnosis, 14*(1), 1–8.

Hilgard, E. R. (1968). *The experience of hypnosis*. New York: Harcourt, Brace, Jovanovich.

Horevitz, R. (1986). Terrifying imagery in hypnosis. In B. Zilbergeld, M. G. Edelstien, & D. L. Araoz (Eds.), *Hypnosis: Questions and answers* (pp. 448–453). New York: Norton.

Hunter, M. (1994). *Creative scripts for hypnotherapy*. New York: Brunner/Mazel.

Ingram, D. H. (1996). The vigor of metaphor in clinical practice. *The American Journal of Psychoanalysis, 56*(1), 17–34.

Jacobs, E., Pelier, E., & Larkin (1998). Ericksonian hypnosis and approaches with pediatric hematology oncology patients. *American Journal of Clinical Hypnosis, 41*(2), 139–154.

Kingsbury, S. (1988). Interacting with trauma. *American Journal of Clinical Hypnosis, 36*(4), 241–247.

Kluft, R. P. (1993). The treatment of dissociative disorder patients: An overview of discoveries, successes, and failures. *Dissociation, 6*, 87–101.

Kohen, D. P., Mann-Rinehard, P., Schmitz, D., & Wills, L. M. (1998). Using hypnosis to help deaf children help themselves: Report of two cases. *American Journal of Clinical Hypnosis, 40*(4), 288–296.

Kroger, W. S. (1963). *Clinical and experimental hypnosis*. Philadelphia: Lippincott.

Lakoff, G., & Johnson, M. (1980). *Metaphors we live by*. Chicago: University of Chicago.

Lankton, S., & Lankton, C. (1986). *Enchantment and intervention in family therapy: Training in Ericksonian approaches*. New York: Brunner/Mazel.

Melville, M. B., & Lykes, M. B. (1992). Guatemalan Indian children and the sociocultural effects of government-sponsored terrorism. *Social Science Medicine, 34*(5), 533–548.

O'Hanlon, W. H. (1987). *Taproots: Underlying principles of Milton Erickson's therapy and hypnosis*. New York: Norton.

Olness, K., & Kohen, D. P. (1996). *Hypnosis and hypnotherapy with children*. New York: Guilford.

Perez, F. (1994). *El vuelo del ave fenix [Flight of the Phoenix]*. Mexico City, Mexico: Editorial Pax Mexico, Libreria Carlos Cesarman, S.A.

Phillips, M. (1993). Turning symptoms into allies: Utilization approaches with posttraumatic symptoms. *American Journal of Clinical Hypnosis, 35*(3), 179–189.

Phillips, M., & Frederick, C. (1995). *Healing the divided self: Clinical and Ericksonian hypnotherapy for posttraumatic and dissociative conditions*. New York: Norton.

Pope, K. S., & Garcia-Peltoniemi, R. E. (1991). Responding to victims of torture: Clinical issues, professional responsibilities, and useful resources. *Professional Psychology: Research and Practice, 22*(4), 269–276.

Robles, T. (1993). *La Magia de Nuestros Disfraces [Magic in the masks we wear].* Mexico City, Mexico: Instituto Milton H. Erickson.

Rosen, S. (Ed). (1982). *My voice will go with you: The teaching tales of Milton H. Erickson.* New York: Norton.

Rossi, E. L. (Ed). (1980). *Collected papers of Milton H. Erickson* (Vols. 1–4). New York: Irvington.

Rossi, E. L., & Cheek, D. (1988). *Mind-body therapy: Methods of ideo-dynamic healing in hypnosis.* New York: Norton.

Siegelman, E. (1990). *Metaphor and meaning in psychotherapy.* New York: Guilford.

Stam, H. J., & Spanos, N. P. (1980). Experimental designs, expectancy effects and hypnotic analgesia. *Journal of Abnormal Psychology, 89*(6), 751–762.

Thompson, K. (1990). Metaphor: A myth with a method. In J. Zeig & S. Gilligan (Eds.), *Brief therapy: Myths, methods and metaphors* (pp. 247–257). New York: Brunner/Mazel.

Voth, H. (1970). The analysis of metaphor. *Journal of the American Psychoanalytic Association, 18*, 599–621.

Wall, V. J. (1988). Hypnosis and children. In D. C. Hammond (Ed.), *Hypnotic suggestion and induction: An introductory manual* (pp. 48–52). Des Plaines, IL: American Society of Clinical Hypnosis.

Wallas, L. (1985). *Stories for the third ear.* New York: Norton.

Watkins, H. H. (1986). Handling a patient who doesn't come out of trance. In B. Zilbergeld, M. G. Edelstien, & D. L. Araoz (Eds.), *Hypnosis: Questions and answers* (pp. 445–447). New York: Norton.

Watkins, J. G., & Watkins, H. H. (1979). The theory and practice of ego-state therapy. In H. Grayson (Ed.), *Short-term approaches to psychotherapy* (pp. 176–220). New York: Wiley.

Watkins, J. G., & Watkins, H. H. (1997). *Ego states: Theory and therapy.* New York: Norton.

Yapko, M. D. (1990). *Trancework.* New York: Brunner/Mazel.

Zahourek, R. P. (1985). *Clinical hypnosis and therapeutic suggestion in nursing*. New York: Grune & Stratton.

Zeig, J. K. (1990). Seeding. In J. K. Zeig & S. Gilligan (Eds.), *Brief therapy: Myths, methods and metaphors* (pp. 163–181). New York: Brunner/Mazel.

Zeig, J. K. (1991). Foreword. In H. Klippstein (Ed.), *Ericksonian hypnotherapeutic group inductions* (p. vii). New York: Brunner/Mazel.

Index

*Capitalized entries in this listing indicate
verbatim inductions and their commen-
taries.